A

TREATISE

ON THE

DISEASES OF FEMALES.

DISORDERS OF MENSTRUATION.

BY JOHN C. PETERS, M. D.

NEW-YORK:
WILLIAM RADDE, No. 322 BROADWAY
PHILADELPHIA: RADEMACHER & SHEEK.—BOSTON: OTIS CLAPP.
ST. LOUIS: J. G. WESSELHOEFT.
LONDON: J. EPPS, 112 GREAT RUSSELL-ST., BLOOMSBURY;
MANCHESTER: TURNER, 41 PICCADILLY.

1854.

Entered according to Act of Congress, in the year 1853, by
WILLIAM RADDE,
In the Clerk's Office of the District Court of the United States for the Southern District of New-York.

POLYGLOT PRINTING OFFICE,
12 Frankfort-st., N. Y.

HOMŒOPATHIC MEDICINES.

WM. RADDE, 322 Broadway, New York, respectfully informs the Homœopathic Physicians, and the friends of the System, that he is the sole Agent for the Leipzig Central Homœopathic Pharmacy, and that he has always on hand a good assortment of the best Homœopathic Medicines, in complete sets or by single vials, in *Tinctures*, *Dilutions* and *Triturations;* also, *Pocket Cases of Medicines; Physicians' and Family Medicine Chests to Laurie's Domestic* (60 to 82 Remedies)—EPP'S (60 Remedies)—HERING'S (60 Remedies to 102).—*Small Pocket Cases* at $3, with Family Guide and 27 Remedies—*Cases* containing 415 vials, with Tinctures and Triturations for Physicians.—*Cases* with 260 Vials of Tinctures and Triturations to Jahr's New Manual, or Symptomen-Codex.—Physicians' *Pocket Cases*, with 60 Vials of Tinctures and Triturations.—*Cases* from 200 to 300 Vials, with low and high dilutions of medicated pellets.—*Cases* from 50 to 80 Vials of low and high dilutions, &c., &c. Homœopathic Chocolate. Refined Sugar of Milk, pure Globules, &c. *Arnica Tincture*, the best specific remedy for bruises, sprains, wounds, &c. *Arnica Plaster*, the best application for *Corns. Urtica urens* and Dr. Reisig's *Homœopathic Pain Extractor* are the best specific remedies for *Burns.* Also, Books, Pamphlets, and Standard Works on the System, in the English, French, and German languages.

HOMŒOPATHIC BOOKS.

JAHR'S NEW MANUAL OF HOMŒOPATHIC PRACTICE; edited, with Annotations, by A. Gerald Hull, M. D. From the last Paris edition. This is the fourth American edition of a very celebrated work, written in French by the eminent Homœopathic Professor Jahr, and it is considered the best practical compendium of this extraordinary science that has yet been composed. After a very judicious and instructive introduction, the work presents a Table of the Homœopathic Medicines, with their names in Latin, English and German; the order in which they are to be studied, with their most important distinctions, and clinical illustrations of their symptoms and effects upon the various organs and functions of the human system. The second volume embraces an elaborate Analysis of the indications in disease, of the medicines adapted to cure, and a Glossary of the technics used in the work, arranged so luminously as to form an admirable guide to every medical student The whole system is here displayed with a modesty of pretension, and a scrupulosity in statement, well calculated to bespeak candid investigation. This laborious work is indispensable to the students and practitioners of Homœopathy, and highly interesting to medical and scientific men of all classes. Complete Symptomatology and Repertory, 2 vols. bound, $6.

JAHR'S NEW MANUAL: originally published under the name of SYMPTOMEN-CODEX. (Digest of Symptoms.) This work is intended to facilitate a comparison of the parallel symptoms of the various Homœopathic agents, thereby enabling the practitioner to discover the characteristic symptoms of each drug, and to determine with ease and correctness what remedy is most Homœopathic to the existing group of symptoms. Translated with important and extensive additions from various sources, by Charles Julius Hempel, M. D., assisted by James M. Quin, M. D., with revisions and clinical notes by John F. Gray, M. D.; contributions by Drs. A. Gerald Hull, George W. Cook, and Dr. B. F. Joslin of New-York; and Drs. C. Hering, J. Jeanes, C. Neidhard, W. Williamson, and J. Kitchen, of Philadelphia; with a Preface by Constantine Hering, M. D., 2 vols., bound $11

HARTMANN, Dr. FR., DISEASES OF CHILDREN AND THEIR HOMŒOPATHIC TREATMENT. 1853. Bound, $2 00.

☞ This is the most complete work ever written on this subject, containing 514 pages. The learned author's name is a full guarantee for the value of the book to the profession; therefore every physician and lover of science should possess this treasure.

BOOKS BY THE SAME AUTHOR.

ROKYTANSKY'S PATHOLOGICAL ANATOMY; Translated from the German with additions on Diagnosis, from Schönlein, Skoda, and others, by Dr. JOHN C. PETERS. 75 cents.

Opinions of the Press.—"Dr. Rokytansky's book is no more than it professes to be: it is morbid Anatomy in its densest and most compact form, scarcely ever alleviated by histories, cases, or hypotheses. It is just such a work as might be expected from its author, who is said to have written in it the result of his experience gained in the careful examination of over 12,000 bodies, and who is possessed of a truly marvellous power of observing and amassing facts. In the course of our analysis we have said comparatively little of its merits, the best evidence of which is found in the length to which our abstracts have been carried without passing beyond the bounds of what is novel or important. Nor would this fault have been committted though much more had been borrowed, for no modern volume on morbid Anatomy contains half so many genuine facts as this; it is alone sufficient to place its author in the highest rank of European medical observers."—*British and Foreign Medical Review.*

Just Published:

RUECKERT, TH. J., A TREATISE ON HEADACHES; with Introduction, Appendix, Synopsis, Notes, Directions for Doses, and eighty additional cases, by JOHN C. PETERS, M. D. 1853. Bound. 75 cents.

"Dr. Peters' book owes its existence to the work of Dr. Rückert just alluded to, but it is no mere translation, indeed it may almost be considered as an original and independent treatise on Headaches. To a certain extent the author has followed Rückert's arrangement, and given all his cases and clinical remarks, but Dr. Peters' volume is enriched by more than eighty additional cases taken from sources not accessible to Rückert, to wit, the French, English and American homœopathic publications. Scattered throughout the work are many useful practical remarks in the form of notes, and at the end is a good synopsis of the indications for the employment of the different remedies for headache. There is also an excellent introductory chapter on the nature and causes of headaches, which contains much curious and interesting information. We may give the reader some notion of the immense amount of original matter in Dr. Peters' volume, when we state that the number of pages in Rückert's work occupied by headaches is but 68, whereas Dr. Peters' book contains 173 pages of nearly equal size.

"Dr. Peters promises a second volume, on Apoplexy, encephalitis, and hydrocephalus, still founded, we presume, on the work of Rückert; and if he shall follow Rückert through all his diseases in the manner in which this volume is executed, we shall be forced to admit that the German original has, like a bishop, gained by translation."—*British Journal of Homœopathy.*

RUECKERT ON APOPLEXY AND PALSY. Successful Homœopathic Cures, collected from the best homœopathic periodicals. Translated and edited by J. C. PETERS, M. D. With full descriptions of the dose to each single case. 1853. Bound, 75 cts.

A TREATISE ON THE DISEASES OF FEMALES—commencing with the Disorders of Menstruation—by JOHN C. PETERS, M. D., with full description of the dose to each single case. 1853. Bound, 75 cts.

In Press:

A TREATISE ON THE DISEASES OF MARRIED FEMALES, including the Disorders of Pregnancy, Parturition, and Lactation, by J. C. PETERS, M. D.

Preparing for Press:

A TREATISE ON THE DISEASES OF THE WOMB, OVARIES, AND UTERINE APPENDAGES—by JOHN C. PETERS, M. D.

N. B.—A Treatise on Diseases of the Eye and Ear, and one on Nervous Diseases and Mental Derangements, are ready for publication.

AUTHOR'S PREFACE.

DURING the last few years the Diseases of Women have excited unusual attention among homœopathic physicians; the labors of Williamson, Madden, Leadam, Croserio, Loomis, Griesselich, Hering, Hartmann, Marcy and Humphreys need only be alluded to in proof of this.

More than a year ago I had engaged to re-publish and edit Leadam's work on the Diseases of Females; but several reasons, the most potent of which was want of time, obliged me to postpone my intentions. A few months ago, my publisher urged me so strongly to publish that I did not feel at liberty to decline; and within a week after, the first instalment of copy was placed in the printer's hands. I have been enabled to keep pace with the demands of "printer's devils" by the aid of the extended preparations which were made a year ago, but especially by the aid of numerous notes upon almost every disease, and upon the action of almost every remedy, which I have patiently been accumulating during the course of twelve or fifteen years. The gaps in my knowledge have been filled up by diligent recourse to the best works and periodicals, both homœopathic and allopathic—American, English, French, and German. Among these, the works of Roberton, Whitehead, Ashwell, Colombat, Churchill, Tilt, Beauvais, Malaise, Rückert, Henderson, Leadam, Trousseau, Valliex, Ranking, Braithwaite, the British Journal of Homœopathy, &c., have been most frequently in my hands. I believe I have always indicated the source from which I have obtained my materials; but wish to state here, once for all, that I much prefer merely transcribing the exact words of an author, to stealing his thoughts and dressing them up in better or worse English than his own. I had intended to make some severe remarks as to the course pursued by Leadam and others in this respect, but as I have frequently availed myself of their pains-taking compilations, I will leave that unpleasant task to others.

This brochure will be quickly followed by another on the Diseases of Married Females, and that by a third, upon the Organic Diseases of the Womb and Ovaries.

J. C. PETERS.

742 Broadway, New-York.

To the Memory

OF

CALEB TICKNOR, A.M., M.D.,

LATE PROFESSOR OF HYGIENE IN THE UNIVERSITY OF THE CITY OF NEW-YORK;

AUTHOR OF

THE PHILOSOPHY OF LIVING; A GUIDE FOR MOTHERS; AN EXPOSITION OF QUACKERY AND IMPOSTURE IN MEDICINE; A PHILOSOPHY OF MEDICINE.

BORN IN SALISBURY, A. D. 1804.

Died in New-York, September, 1840, æt. 36.

"Distinguished for his love of study and investigation, sacred regard for truth, his frank and fearless spirit in the avowal of matured opinions, honorable and gentlemanly deportment, affectionate and kindly disposition, elevated but humble christian character.

"A man of fine accomplishments, but of finer dispositions; of goodly distinction, but of better promise; of ardent earthly hopes in this life, but of stronger heavenly hopes in his death."—Rev. Adam Reid.

"Dr. Ticknor was extensively known in this country and in Europe. His 'Philosophy of Living' gave him a reputation wherever the English language is spoken. He was talented, industrious and philanthrophic, and devoted to the science of Medicine because it gave him an opportunity of doing good. He became a thorough convert to Homœopathy, from an honest conviction that it was a rational system, notwithstanding the ridicule it so often excites. The idea of profiting by what is usually considered a hallucination of a portion of the civilized world, never once entered his mind. He was honest in his intentions, and dared to brave the public sentiment which at one time set with a strong flood against him. We esteemed him for his integrity and sterling worth and character, and now mourn his early death as an irreparable loss to the republic of letters, to science, and to humanity."—J. V. C. Smith, M. D., *Ed. Boston Med. and Surg. Journal.*

ON THE

NATURE AND CAUSES

OF

MENSTRUATION.

ON PUBERTY AND FIRST MENSTRUATION.

ON PUBERTY.

This period in the female may be defined as that in which the girl fully commences that general growth and development of all her organs, which renders her a young woman, and receives those functions which makes her fit to be a wife, and capable of becoming a mother.

Evidences of the changes which mark the advent of puberty, are often detected many months and sometimes years, before it is fully accomplished; but more commonly, up to a short time before puberty, we notice only the natural, but proportionably more rapid growth of the whole body, to such an extent, that the stature and size of the majority of girls is nearly attained before the crisis is fully accomplished. But at the period of puberty, growth and development receive a still more rapid impulse, and the lank figure and unrestrained movements of the awkward girl, are changed in the short space of a few months, into the finished form, reserved manners, and graceful deportment of conscious womanhood.

The age of puberty ought to be distinguished by changes in the character of the girl, fully as extensive as those of the *physique*. The nervous system should show unusual sensibility and susceptibility; the mind should acquire more extended powers of emotion and passion, and the imagination become more lively and animated. The pelvic viscera should become rapidly developed, and the hips enlarged; the breasts should become rounded and full, and establish their sympathy with the womb; the chest, throat and arms should acquire the contour of a maturer development, and the whole body become more rounded, full and adipose; the hair should grow more luxuriantly, the skin become fresh and blooming, the voice full and mellow, and the whole female figure should acquire that elegance of symmetry, the complexion that bloom of health and beauty, and each feature and action that play of intellect and emotion, and that indescribable gracefulness of action, which are to be found united in woman alone.—WHITEHEAD.

It is evident that when all these changes are absent, or imperfectly accomplished, that although ordinary dietetic and hygienic means, aided by common nervines and tonics, &c., may help somewhat, still, such is the intricacy and beauty of the whole natural process, that more subtle and sympathetic means are required. All these external changes and developments are attended with, or even dependent upon similar internal ones, especially in the ovaries and uterus. The ovaries in particular become more active. These organs, it is well known, contain certain bodies called Graafian vesicles, which in their turn enclose the true ova or germs of future human beings, first accurately described by De Baer, and hence called ovules of De Baer. Before puberty, the Graafian vesicles are scarcely visible, but about the tenth year of life, a whitish or grayish pulpy substance is deposited in them, and when this changes to a yellow color, from the deposit of a yellow, brain-like granular substance, so much like the ordinary substance of the brain and nerves, as to be scarcely distinguished from it, then the first signs of puberty become manifest in the girl; the ovules of De Baer become more and more developed, and before each monthly period, one Graafian vesicle commences to increase very greatly in size, until at the menstrual period it forms a tumor on the surface of the one or the other ovary, about the size of a small nut, or medium cherry, having increased in a few days from an infinitesimal body, only one-half, or at the very most three lines in diameter, to the above dimensions. From this time forward, at each monthly period, one Graafian vesicle and its contained De Baer's ovule, successively arrives at maturity, approaches the surface and lacerates the capsule of the ovary, is then grasped by the fimbriated extremities of the Fallopian tubes, and is finally conveyed along to the womb. Simultaneously with this increase of action in the ovaries, the womb also becomes the seat of greater nervous and vascular activity, accompanied with congestion of blood to, and pouring out of the menstrual fluid from its internal surface. The periodical monthly returns of ovarian activity and congestion, tend to the growth, development and expulsion into the womb of ovules, or germs of future human beings, one of which is sacrificed at each menstrual period, unless conception take place. The simultaneous periodic activity, and congestion of the womb tends to the production of the envelopes or membranes which would enshroud the germ, and if conception take place, to the proper supply of it with blood and nutriment, or materials for growth. Hence, shortly before, or after the menstrual flow, is the only period of time when vivification of the germ can take place; the exceptions to this rule, according to Raciborski, do not exceed six or seven per cent.*

The rapid development of the Graafian vesicles, from their rudimentary state to the required menstrual size, causes pressure upon the body of the ovary and its aroused vessels and nerves, in like manner as the growth and development of a tooth presses aside and stretches the substance of the gums in a child, causing comparable local pains, and more or less distant sympathetic derangement in both processes. Nervousness, restlessness, pain about the groin, or ovary which is

* In almost all cases of recent menstruation in which death took place accidentally, by sickness, or by hanging, in which menstruation had but just commenced, the substance of the ovaries, tubes and cornuæ of the uterus, quite near the insertion of the tubes, have been found most congested—proving, apparently, that the menstrual excitement and congestion commences in the ovaries, passes next to the tubes, and then encroaches gradually upon the uterus, progressing from the neighborhood of the tubes downwards.

the seat of the process, pains and derangement in the back, hips, stomach, bowels, headaches, colics, diarrhœas, and even convulsions may attend the process.

Prior to, and during each catamenial period, the mammæ sympathize with the uterus—the breasts become swollen and tender, and a degree of irritability in the whole organ exists. As the menstrual flow sets in, these symptoms disappear, and the breasts either resume their former state and size, or they become slightly diminished, especially as age advances, and in the unmarried state.

But the advent of puberty is apt to be attended with an unusual degree of perversion of activity in both the nervous and vascular systems, tending obviously to a state of general excitement and plethora, all of which in due time are relieved by a flow which nature establishes for the purpose. The manners of the changing girl are perceptibly altered, she is disinclined to pursue her accustomed employment and exercises, is languid and listless, often reserved and fretful, her appetite capricious, stomach and bowels disturbed, sleep irregular and unrefreshing;—pain in the back and head, and weight, fulness, heat, and some irritation of lower part of abdomen, are also apt to occur.

But very often these symptoms are short and transitory, or even absent altogether, and the flow sets in more or less scantily or freely, being either at first thin, serous or mucous, colorless or but slightly colored, and after continuing a few days, subsides, and health and comfort are speedily restored. At each succeeding period the flow presents more of the normal red appearance, which it finally acquires in full, after several repetitions of the process.

But it is not always that puberty advances thus gradually and progressively, and it would always be well for the mother, whenever she perceives any of these indications, to lose no time in preparing her daughter to expect the change which is the common lot of her sex, so that the first appearance of the menstrual flow may neither be arrested by the alarm naturally felt at something hitherto inexperienced, nor by the dangerous applications to which in her ignorance she may imprudently have recourse.

To prove the necessity of this preparatory caution on the part of the mother, TILT found that out of 100 girls, 25 were unprepared for its appearance; 13 out of the 25 were much frightened, screamed, or went into hysterics; and 6 out of the 13 thought themselves injured, and attempted to stop the flow with cold water. Of those much frightened, the flow was checked by the mental emotion in 7 instances, and never restored in 3, while the general health of all was seriously impaired. Of the six who washed in cold water, 2 succeeded in effectually stopping the flow, which only reappeared after several years, and then at irregular intervals, and was never healthily reëstablished.

It will readily happen to all but very thoughtful mothers, that the first menstruation may make its appearance before her daughter has been forewarned. But when the monthly flow has once occurred, it is imperatively necessary that right advice and information should be given to the child; for many girls view the whole matter with such strong disgust and levity, that they expose themselves carelessly or purposely at the regular term, to cold and wet, or use cold baths or other means of suppression, finally bringing on disordered menstruation, and permanent ill-health, by thus trifling with the function, in the same way that a child plays with a watch, setting the hands backwards and forwards to amuse and injure themselves. The mother should institute a monthly regimen—keep an exact account of dates and particulars—prevent all unusual exposure for a few days before the expected flow, such as to night air, damp linen, thin dresses, wet feet, cold and acid drinks, balls and entertainments, when practicable. When the "custom of women" has been fully and regularly established, such extreme precautions are of course not only unnecessary, but in many cases unadvisable.

Thoughtless mothers will always allow their daughters to be taken unawares, but even the most thoughtful may be forestalled. Menstruation may set in for the first time from a severe fall, violent jumping, great mental emotion, or an extraordinarily long walk—and in such cases, TILT says there may be a considerable flow in 30 per cent., while in 8 per cent. it may amount to absolute flooding, lasting from 8 to 10 days, and requiring medical treatment. These facts are important, because they are not in accordance with the general belief, and if duly acquainted with them, the mother, in such sudden and extreme cases, will not only maintain her own composure, but impart it to those around her, and reassure her daughter that nothing has happened but what is not exceedingly uncommon, and easily to be remedied by rest in the horizontal posture, cool drinks, light covering in cool and well ventilated apartments, with the aid of a few drops of Tinct. Cinnamon, &c., until medical advice can be obtained.

At other times, or rather in other cases, the occurrence of Menstruation may be long protracted—excessive languor, drowsiness, violent pain in the head, or along the spine, and around the lower part of stomach and bowels, may alternate with rigors and feverish reaction, or with nervous symptoms, and even spasms; clearly indicating a loss of balance between the circulatory and nervous systems, which if not timely remedied, may lead to very injurious consequences—to violent congestions, or inflammations; or to scrofulous disease of some important organ, if there be a hereditary tendency that way; or to various nervous, spasmodic, or painful affections, when the nervous system predominates. Aconite and Hyosciamus are the most important remedies here, although Stramonium may be required.

In another class of women, previous to the first appearance of the menses and during their flow, the venous, biliary or lymphatic systems may be deranged—the face assumes a sallow, greenish, yellowish or bloated pasty look, the eyes are dull and sunken, or surrounded by a dark areola, which appearances are present ever afterwards in a greater or less degree, during every monthly flow, the result of functional difficulty at the commencement, and generally dependent upon and associated with a languid circulation through the venous and portal systems, and a low nervous power.—WHITEHEAD. Conium, Pulsatilla, Manganese, Colchicum, &c., will often be required.

If the changes at puberty be well accomplished, such is the intensity of vitality, and the impulse given to every nerve and organ, that the system resists all baneful influences, and sickness and death are less frequent at this period of life than any other. But on the other hand, original delicacy of constitution, or carelessness, will render this period preëminently favorable to the propagation of new forms of disease, or to the development of those latent germs of disorder which have existed from birth. Hence, the first appearancc of the menses should be watched for with some care and anxiety on the part of the mother.

ON FIRST MENSTRUATION.

IN order to have exact data for any opinions which may be here advanced, I have with some little labor collected the largest table of the periods of first Menstruation that has ever been published, viz., of 29,918 women, observed by Du Boismont, Bennett, Lee, Whitehead, Roberton, Tilt, &c., &c.

1. In one case, in an infant, the flow commenced a few days after birth, and continued regular at periods of 3 weeks, till her death at the age of 4 years and some months, at which time she was developed in size and figure, like a girl of 10 or 11 years.

2. Of these, there is one case in which a child menstruated at 9 months of age, and continued regular subsequently.

3. Also, one case of a child born with signs of puberty, who menstruated for the first time at 3 years of age, and continued regular.

1 case menstruated at 4½ years of age.
1 " at 5 years of age.
1 " " 7 " "

2	cases	at	8 years of age.
20	"	"	9 " "
92	"	"	10 " "
125	"	"	from 10 to 11 years.
278	"	"	11 years.
399	"	"	from 11 to 12 years.
495	"	"	12 years.
656	"	"	from 12 to 13 years.
852	"	"	13 years.
934	"	"	from 13 to 14 years.
1417	"	"	14 years.
1562	"	"	from 14 to 15 years.
1659	"	"	15 years.
2048	"	"	from 15 to 16 years.
1634	"	"	16 years.
1792	"	"	from 16 to 17 years.
793	"	"	17 years.
1397	"	"	from 17 to 18 years.
761	"	"	18 years.
1023	"	"	from 18 to 19 years.
326	"	"	19 years.
591	"	"	from 19 to 20 years.
170	"	"	20 years.
379	"	"	from 20 to 21 years.
14	"	"	21 years.
148	"	"	from 21 to 22 years.
29	"	"	22 years.
90	"	"	from 22 to 23 years.
9	"	"	23 years.
36	"	"	from 23 to 24 years.
3	"	"	24 years.
15	"	"	from 24 to 25 years.
4	"	"	from 25 to 26 years.
5	"	"	from 26 to 27 years.
1	"	"	from 29 to 30 years.

But the above table was compiled from cases taken in all climates, hot, cold, and temperate, and hence is not a sufficient guide for the inhabitants of either. Of the 29,918 cases, 766 occurred in hot climates, 6745 in cold, and 15,154 in temperate climates.

At YEARS.	766 Cases HOT.	6745 Cases, COLD.	16,154 Cases, TEMPERATE.	At YEARS.
5	0	0	1	5
7	0	0	1	7
8	0	0	2	8
9	3	0	16	9
10	9	0	83	10
11	21	1	481	11
12	96	5	783	12
13	159	19	1360	13
14	133	113	2105	14
15	103	372	2675	15
16	55	738	2869	16
17	39	741	1795	17
18	26	615	1497	18
19	10	540	799	19
20	8	360	393	20
21	2	278	126	21
22	2	114	43	22
23	1	73	22	23
24	2	27	11	24
25	0	12	3	25
26	0	4	2	26
27	0	5	0	27
30	0	1	0	30

Several very important facts may be adduced from the above table, viz.: the hastening effect of heat, the retarding effect of cold, and the great number of both precocious and tardy cases which occur in all climates. Many a consumptive parent is sent to the South merely to die; many a non-menstruating girl might be sent there to live; many a woman with profuse Menstruation might be restored to health by a season spent at the North. The table also corroborates the well known necessity for warmth of clothing and residence, for those with scanty Menstruation, and *vice versa*. Menstruation occurs in the daughters of the rich, 9 months before it does in those of the working classes placed in the most comfortable circumstances, and 14 months before its average appearance in the poorest classes. It should also be borne in mind that the season of the year at which the girl becomes of the proper age, has a great influence upon the first appearance, almost as much as hereditary influence; women of the frozen regions, as the Samoiedes lose but a very small quantity of blood, and that in the summer season only, while the Greenlanders have scarcely any discharge on account of the cold. On the other hand, it is quite certain that European women who migrate to a hotter climate, such as that of the West and East Indies, often perish in consequence of the excessive menstrual losses, and their great liability to abortion with hæmorrhage.

It is evident from the second table, that the majority of women in *hot* climates reach the age of puberty and menstruate between the 12th and 15th years of age; in *temperate* climates between the 13th and 18th years; and in *cold* climates between the 14th and 22d years. We now propose to enter upon an inquiry into the consequences, or advantages and disadvantages of early or late, Menstruation—to determine, as far as possible, when medical aid is required, and when the case may be left to domestic management or to nature. It is satisfactorily established, that, in every country and climate, the period of first Menstruation may be retarded in very many cases much beyond the average age, often without producing ill-health, or the slightest inconvenience. TILT even goes so far as to assume that the great art of managing girls, so as to bring them to the full perfection of womanhood, is to retard the period of Puberty as much as possible.

MANAGEMENT OF FIRST MENSTRUATION.

It is to be taken for granted that every sensible and thoughtful mother will inform her daughter, when signs of Puberty and Menstruation present themselves, of what she is to expect.

According to TILT, during the crisis of Puberty, and until

Puberty is fully confirmed, there should be a general relaxation from study, which might otherwise too forcibly engross the mind, and the energies required by the constitution to work out nature's ends. Even in man, the excess of mental labor is known to produce constipation, by some prostration of the nervous energy; would it not then be likely to have the same effect upon girls—besides tending to check the critical flow which nature contemplates establishing? Nay more, even when puberty is fully confirmed, some days before, and during the time occupied by the monthly function, the head is very often much affected by pain, vertigo, drowsiness, or dulness; in which case the brain should be less severely taxed than usual. Those who are occupied in the education of girls should bear in mind not only this, but also that the same regimen cannot suit all, and that each particular pupil may require a different amount and quality of mental exertion. These precautions are particularly necessary for those girls who have a hereditary, or acquired tendency to sick-headaches; an immense amount of mischief to the head may be brought about by the combined influence of carelessness of the mother to institute a proper monthly regimen for her daughter, and the natural tendency of school teachers to urge on their scholars as much as possible.

Very particular attention should be paid to the clothing of young girls about the menstrual period. Tilt truly says that rich or fashionable young ladies suffer almost as much from insufficient clothing, as the daughters of the absolutely destitute; for poverty and fashion are two inexorable tyrants which exact the same, or similar things, and bring on the same diseases. The feet should be more carefully protected, just before and during the menstrual period; and the upper part of the chest should be less uncovered than most girls are inclined to have it when obliged to go to places of nocturnal amusement.

The mother should take particular care that *the flow be not interrupted, either by carelessness or design.* Of all the causes of suppression, none is so frequently observed as the application of cold and wet to the feet and legs, particularly during the flow, or a few days before, or after its appearance. TILT places much stress upon the effect of draggled clothes in producing this effect; he says in respect to walking, ladies may be divided into three classes:

1st. Those who never raise their dress, but walk through thick and thin, with real or affected indifference to wet and mud.

2d. Those who raise the dress, but allow the mass of under-clothes to collect all the mud, and beat it up to the middle of the leg.

3d. Those who, without offending the rules of propriety and good taste, know how to raise both dress and under-clothes, just sufficiently to protect both.

But suppression occurs almost as frequently from design as from accident; for many mothers, otherwise judicious, will not condescend to give the necessary advice to their daughters, many of whom often attempt to check the discharge by the application of cold water, putting their feet into cold water, &c. They often do this from ignorance, or by the advice of servants, or sisters but little older than themselves. The consequence is, that years may elapse before perfect regularity will be established.

The mother should also be watchful that the function be performed *neither more or less frequently than once a month;* the monthly type is the only type of its healthy performance, and any marked deviation from this rule, rarely coincides with perfect health. Many young girls who would otherwise be quite regular as to time, are exceedingly susceptible to slight influences, so that walking about with their bare feet upon the cold floor in winter, while dressing or undressing; or a walk in the cold air, or a slight chill, will suffice to suppress the discharge instantly. Considerable maternal care, and even authority, should be exerted in these cases. Such girls should not be allowed to go to church or school, in rain or snow storms, much less go to any place of amusement. Volumes might be filled with illustrations of the pernicious effects of the flow being suddenly checked, either intentionally or accidentally. At the monthly period, the uterus, ovaries, and all the branches of the hypogastric, sciatic, and ovaric arteries are full; it is full tide with all that system of vessels; the accompanying nerves are all aroused with the periodical stimulus. The sudden application of cold will produce a spasmodic closure of the excreting orifices of the womb, and the uterus and ovaries instantly become the seat of intense engagement, which will react as a disturbing force upon the whole system, but especially upon any already weakened organ, be that the head, lungs, stomach, or bowels. If the application of cold and wet to merely one part of the body, is capable of producing these bad effects, how much more injurious must be cold bathing at such times, either by the domestic, or professional use of the hydropathic treatment. To advance, in justification of this practice, that cold does not always check the flow, is a shallow excuse, founded on but few exceptional cases, although it is frequently advanced, even when the menses have become habitually scanty, irregular, or painful.—Tilt.

The mother should also be careful that *the pain should not be too violent, or long continued.* Women expect to suffer some pain every month, but the pain need not be intense, protracted, or agonizing. If the sufferings are very considerable, and do not abate with the appearance of the flow, Bellad., Stram., Secale, or Cocculus,* may be used, and if these fail, the medical attendant should be consulted; for, although the belief prevails, that because the function is a natural one, all its attendant pains must be endured, so little is this true, that the frequent occurrence of severe pain is almost proof positive of carelessness, either upon the part of the mother or daughter, or both. The severe pains are very generally rheumatic in their nature, and originate and are kept up by the exciting causes of rheumatism, viz., insufficient clothing of the person or feet, or thoughtless exposure to cold and wet.

The mother should also be watchful *that the flow be not too*

* Full directions for the *doses* of all these remedies will be given subsequently.

abundant, or of too long coutinuance. Tilt says there is another deep-rooted and most dangerous prejudice, which makes women believe that, however great may be the discharge, if it occur regularly, it is in perfect accordance with the views of nature. He has frequently drawn a parent's attention to the debility and ill health following an habitually too copious flow, and as frequently received the same answer, "She is always so;" so difficult is it to enforce the conviction that the fact of a girl *being always so*, is the very reason for adopting such measures as should prevent her ever being so.

The monthly flow must not be accompanied by too much mucous discharge, commonly known by the name of "the whites." Although the regular establishment of Menstruation is generally and naturally preceded and followed, for a day or two, by a white discharge, which must be considered a part of its phenomena, still, if this discharge becomes excessive, or too long continued, or instead of being white and unaccompanied with pain, changes to yellow or green, and is attended with much pain in the back and thighs,—then it becomes a disorder requiring medical interference. Sabina, Copaiba, Bovista, and other remedies, may be required.

The monthly function should not be attended by much hysteria, or severe nervous symptoms. The most frequent of all nervous symptoms of this function, is a peculiar affection of the head, not amounting to actual pain, or sick-headache, or hysterics, but easily aggravated into one or the other of these, if excessive exertions of body or mind be enforced; it is a dull, heavy, stupid feeling, with a great tendency to sleep; it varies from a slight heaviness, to variable shades of severity, which may become much aggravated by worry or anxiety of mind, by struggling to learn long and stupid lessons, in order to satisfy some exacting school-teacher, or to retain some post of honor in a class. Girls affected decidedly in this way, should be treated with great leniency, and even indulgence, at each monthly period.

The tendency to diarrhœa should not be too decided. More or less tendency to looseness of the bowels is almost natural at the monthly period, but it should not be so excessive as to diminish the quantity of the flow, much less to take its place. In 449 cases, collected by BUTLER LANE and TILT, this "catamenial diarrhœa" occurred in 189 instances, so that more or less of this symptom may be expected in about half of all cases. If it be excessive, Veratrum, Aloes, or Bryonia may be required. For *dose*, see subsequently.

But the most important point of all is, that mothers should undertake and carry out a system of judicious supervision of the health, diet, exercise, clothing, habits, &c., of changing girls.

REGULAR MENSTRUATION.

1. TIME OF FIRST OCCURRENCE.

From 14 to 16 years of age is by far the most regular and common time for first menstruation to set in, in temperate climates. In a table compiled from the cases collected by WHITEHEAD, DE BOISMONT, LEE, BENNETT, &c., consisting of 8489 cases, more than one half, or 4689, commenced during these years, viz.:

1417 cases at 14 years.
1658 " 15 "
1614 " 16 ".

In another collection of cases by TILT, of 15,154 young women, no less than 7649 cases, or rather more than one-half, also commenced to menstruate between their 14th and 15th years, viz.:

2105 cases at 14 years.
2675 " 15 "
2869 " 16 "

According to WHITEHEAD, this period, from 14 to 16 years of age, is not only the most regular and common age for Menstruation to commence in temperate climates, but is also almost necessarily the most favorable; for of 1728 cases occurring during these years, and observed by himself, only about 324 were attended with unusual, painful, or unfavorable symptoms—or only about 19 per cent. The percentage of irregular, difficult, or unfavorable cases, among the precocious and tardy, is much higher, ranging from 22 to 47 per cent.

The occurrence of Menstruation one or two years before 14, or at 13 and 12 years, and also one or two years later than 16, i. e., at 17 or 18, is not sufficiently uncommon to be regarded as decidedly irregular, although the former is rather too early, and the latter decidedly too late. Of the 23,643 cases in the two tables above quoted, as many as 8356, or about one-third set in at the 12th or 13th, or 17th or 18th years, viz.:

1379	cases	at 12	years.
2212	"	13	"
2578	"	17	"
2188	"	18	"

All cases of Menstruation occurring for the first time before the 12th year, or after the 18th, must be regarded as very decidedly precocious, or tardy.

2. TIME OF RECURRENCE.

In regular Menstruation, the flow should return every lunar month, or every 28 days, counting from the beginning of one period to the commencement of the next, leaving a free period of 23 or 24 days, and including a flow of four or five days' continuance, thus completing the four lunar weeks or 28 days. Roberton, of Manchester, thinks that only about 61 women out of every hundred are thus regular to the true time of 28 days, calculating from a table of 450 cases. Condie, of Philadelphia, basing his opinion on 784 cases, thinks that 71 women out of every hundred, have an interval between the cessation of the flow of one period and its recurrence at the next, of 28 days, scarcely ever deviating, and then only in a few cases, for a single day, or at most two days, either anticipating or postponing. Tilt, from 100 cases, makes the average of perfectly regular women as high as 77 out of every hundred. Roberton, of Manchester, out of 520 cases, found 324 who had a regular interval of a lunar month.

Slight variations from this normal standard must not be regarded as unnatural, as cases are met with in perfectly healthy women, in whom the monthly flow occurs with the utmost regularity, every 25, 26 or 27 days, instead of every 28. WHITEHEAD, in 520 cases, found about 35 women who were regularly unwell at intervals varying from 20 to 27 days; but whatever the interval, whether 20 or 25 days, or more, it had always been the same in the same person.

Again, in 51 cases, WHITEHEAD noticed that, although Menstruation set in every 28 days, still, every 3d or 4th month, a difference of 3 or more days was observed in the duration of the discharge, coupled with an increase in quantity.

In 38 other cases, the menses recurred every lunar month as a rule, but set in every 3d or 4th month from 4 to 7 days earlier; and these regular deviations were so marked and constant in most instances, as to be expected and anticipated by preparations for them, at the particular times.

In 14 cases, the interval was only 24 days, but occasionally prolonged to 28 days.

One lady menstruated regularly every 28 days, but at the middle of every 3d month, she had an intercurrent discharge, lasting from 30 to 40 hours.

In another case, Menstruation generally occurred every 28 days, but every 3d month she missed one period, thus having a free interval of 2 months, her health never suffering in consequence.

From the frequency of such cases, WHITEHEAD says, some writers have assumed that the menstrual discharge is augmented periodically and naturally, every 2d, 3d or 4th month. ARISTOTLE believed that such an increase took place regularly every 3d month. A knowledge of these variations is of importance, as they are often the occasion of considerable, though perhaps unnecessary anxiety, and frequently much harm is done by premature medical or domestic interference, thus perverting a means which nature had intended to act beneficially.

The regularity of the recurrence of Menstruation is supposed, by RACIBORSKI, to depend entirely upon the regular growth, maturation, and periodical discharge of the ova. That these, like the seeds and eggs of vegetables, insects, and birds have a certain definite and regular period allowed for their formation and ripening. That the development of Graafian vesicles, or ova, ought to be considered not merely as the cause of Menstruation, but the essential and most important part of it; and that a woman may regularly develope her ova and be liable to conceive, even when she may never have had the outward and visible signs of her catamenia.

GALL, whilst not admitting a sidereal influence, believed that the discharge would be found generally to take place at about the same period of time, and that there are certain weeks in each month in which few or no women are menstruating. He divides the menstrual epochs into two classes, comprising the first 8 days of the 1st and 2d fortnight, i. e., the 1st and 3d weeks of each lunar month. GALL even insists that those women who, from accidental causes, become *unwell* during the 2d and 4th weeks, will soon return under the influence of the general law. However this may be, every physician in large practice will often find a large number of women menstruating about the same time.

3. REGULARITY AS TO DURATION.

The most common and regular length of time for the menstrual flow to continue, is from 4 to 6 days. A flow which lasts only 3 days or less, must be regarded as rather short, while one which lasts 7, 8, or 9 days or more, is decidedly too prolonged, although it may not prove injurious to some individuals.

4. REGULARITY AS TO QUANTITY.

This is much more difficult to determine than one would

suppose. BOUCHARDAT had one case in which 1 ounce flowed every 10 hours, by measurement, making about 12 ounces in 120 hours, or 5 days. MEIGS, of Philadelphia, is confident that many healthy women lose 2 or 3 ounces per day, for from 5 to 7 days, amounting in all to 10 or 15, or even 20 ounces per term. But these conclusions are undoubtedly much above the general average. WHITEHEAD, of Manchester, calculates 4, 6, or 9 ounces, as the general average in temperate climates. BAUDELOCQUE thought that most French women lose only from 3 or 4, to 6 ounces. In Holland, the average is placed at 6 ounces; in Germany, at 6, 8 or 12 ounces; in Spain, at 14 or 15 ounces; in Greece, at 18 or 20 ounces, &c. It is probable that 6 or 8 ounces is the normal standard—although 4 or 5 ounces per term may not be too little for some persons, nor 10 12, or a few ounces more, too much for others. MEIGS, of Philadelphia, thinks the quantity may vary normally from a few ounces to 20, or more. He has repeatedly inquired the number of changes of napkins required in the whole period of 5 or 7 days, and has often been informed that some women change twice, or thrice, or even four times in 24 hours. Now three changes per day, for 7 days, will give 21 napkins, on each of which are found at least 2 tablespoonfuls of blood, at which estimate we shall have the result of 21 ounces for the whole product; and he is confident that many healthy women lose fully this quantity, as the regular and natural elimination. LOOMIS estimates the normal quantity as low as from 2 to 4 ounces.

5. REGULARITY AS TO QUALITY.

Normal menstrual blood has an acid reaction, while systemic blood is always alkaline. RETZIUS, of Stockholm, has discovered free phosphoric and lactic acids in the menstrual discharge. It is well known that menstrual blood does not coagulate like ordinary blood, and it has been demonstrated, that the addition of a small quantity of acetic, lactic or phosphoric acid, or of almost any other acid to natural blood will prevent it from coagulating, and approximate it in properties, and appearance to menstrual blood. The acid seems to act by dissolving the free, or uncombined fibrin contained in systemic blood.

It has long been a mooted point, whether menstrual blood is a true secretion, or simply an exudation of pure blood. WHITEHEAD decides in favor of the latter supposition ; he insists that true menstrual blood, uncombined with the normally acid vaginal mucus, is like ordinary blood, and equally capable of coagulation ; but that it is immediately dissolved in the vaginal mucus, being thus enabled to pass off in an uninterrupted stream. Here is observed, he says, one of those most wise and merciful provisions of the great Creator and Preserver of all things, which so frequently strike the physiologist with wonder and admiration. If no such solvent power as that of the acid vaginal mucus existed, the coagulated part of the menstrual secretion, being, on account of its consistence, necessarily more or less detained within the vaginal canal, would soon become a mass of dead and putrid animal matter, and the consequences would be awful in the extreme.

IRREGULAR MENSTRUATION.

In its largest sense, this includes all departures from the natural standard, whether Menstruation be unusually early or late in the time of its first appearance ; or recurs at too short or too long intervals of time, viz., as often as every 2 or 3 weeks, or less ; or only every 5 or 6 weeks, or more ; or lasts too short a time, viz., less than 3 or 4 days, or continues too long, viz., as much as 6, 8, 10, or 14 days, or more ; being attended with too scanty a flow, viz., only 1, 2, or more ounces, or with too profuse a discharge, viz., more than 8, 10, 12, or 20, or more ounces ; or being preceded, accompanied, or followed by severe pain, distress, or other unusual circumstances. In its more common sense, it refers merely to those cases in which Menstruation recurs at irregular, and indeterminate periods of time.

Of the 8,489 cases already alluded to, about 20 cases were

exceedingly and irregularly precocious, Menstruation occurring from a few days, to a few months after birth; or at three or five years of age, or at eight or nine years. About 50 cases were decidedly and irregularly *late* in the period of first occurrence, viz., as late as 21, or 26 years of age.

Of 5,547 cases collected by WHITEHEAD, DE BOISMONT and BENNETT, no less than 1,742 accomplished the changes of puberty with more or less irregularity, as far as regards suffering, delay or difficulty, each monthly return being attended with pain or discomfort of some kind, or with scanty or profuse discharge, or occurring at irregular intervals of time.

In 1,404 cases, in which particular attention was paid to the time of the recurrence of Menstruation, by ROBERTON, CONDIE, and WHITEHEAD, no less than 463 females were found to be irregular as to time. In 1,045 cases, 96 had returns every three weeks regularly; 134 women were unwell every 14 days; and 89 were so extremely irregular as to afford no means of calculating the periods of recurrence, the duration, or quantity of the discharge.

ROBERTON, of Manchester, thinks that only in 61 per cent. of cases does Menstruation recur regularly and monthly, viz., with a free interval of 23 or 24 days, and a flow of 4 or 5 days, completing a period of 4 weeks, or 28 days. He also thinks that there is another large class of women amounting to 28 per cent. of the whole number, in whom the natural term is only 3 weeks; in another and smaller class, embracing about 10 per cent. in number, the returns are irregular and uncertain, but in his opinion not from the effect of disease, the term varying in length from 4, or 6, or 8, to even 12 weeks. In a fourth, but much smaller class of cases, the menses return regularly and normally, for the class, as often as every fortnight, the free interval being only 9 or 10 days, the flow lasting 4 or 5 days each time, or 8 or 10 days out of every month.

CONDIE, of Philadelphia, speaks still more decidedly on these points; he insists that, in about 71 per cent., the interval between the cessation of the flow and its recurrence amounts to 28 days, never deviating, and that in a few cases only, beyond a single day, or 2 days. In about 18 per cent. he found that the menses returned at intervals of very nearly 21 days, but in many cases the flow at each alternate period was much more copious, and lasted for a day or two longer; all these women were in the enjoyment of perfect health, although they feared that the frequent recurrence of the discharge was the result of disease, or was calculated to weaken them. CONDIE says, that, after the most minute investigation, he was satisfied that their fears were unfounded. In about 5 per cent. of CONDIE's cases, the menses returned every 2 weeks; in about 6 per cent. at very irregular and uncertain periods, varying from 2 to 8, or 10 weeks, all generally occurring in females of relaxed and excitable constitutions, several being affected with dyspepsia, hysteria, or leucorrhœa.

WHITEHEAD's general experience has already been quoted (see p. 17). TILT assumes, that about 77 per cent. of all women are perfectly regular; about 19 per cent. have too frequent returns, viz., as often as every 3 weeks; and that only about 5 per cent. are exceedingly irregular and uncertain.

In 9 cases out of 359, Menstruation lasted only one day each time; in 15 cases out of 161, the menses set in every 3 weeks as a rule, but every third or fourth return occurred from 4 to 7 days later; in 14 cases out of 161, the interval was usually 24 days, but occasionally 28 days; in 5 cases the returns happened every 5 or 6 weeks, but occasionally every 4 weeks; in 2 cases Menstruation recurred every 18 days generally, but an interval of a month was interposed every third or fourth period; one lady menstruated every 28 days, but at the middle of every third interval, she had an intercurrent discharge, lasting 30 or 40 hours; finally, in 32 cases out of 161, the returns were so irregular as to afford no means of calculating either the recurrence, duration, or quantity.

TREATMENT OF IRREGULAR MENSTRUATION.

TILT insists, that the periods may often be rendered perfectly regular as to time, by the careful use of Quinine. Veratrum, Staphysagria, Phosphoric acid, Mercurius acet., and Nux vomica are supposed to possess the power of restoring irregular Menstruation to a regular recurrence at the time of every new moon; if this be so, it would be advisable to pay particular attention to the administration of these remedies just before the time of the new moon. Sulphur and Ruta are regarded as the most homœopathic remedies for very irregular Menstruation. Manganum aceticum is also homœopathic when the menses are apt to recur at unusual periods.

Dose.—The use of these remedies should be commenced at least 2 weeks before the full moon: Of *Veratrum*, Noack advises 1 or 2 drop doses of the 2d, 3d, 6th, or 12th dilution, once or twice a day; or from 3 to 5 granules may be given night and morning; the same doses of Staphysagria, Nux vomica, and Ruta may be used. One or two grains per dose of the powder of Phosphoric acid, Mercurius acet., or of Manganum acet., may be given every 2d night for one week; then every night for the next three days, and every night and morning for the 3 days just preceding the new moon; the 1st, 3d, 6th, or 12th trituration may be given, or from 3 to 5 granules per dose.

PRECOCIOUS MENSTRUATION.

A precocious puberty is generally observed in girls possessing the sanguine temperament, and in those who exhibit a delicate organization of structure. Although the contrary has been supposed, Colombat justly says that "Observation proves, that women in whom the nervous temperament predominates, are regulated both sooner and more copiously than others; and that all the causes which exalt this temperament, such as powerful passions, culture of the arts, and amusements, light reading, &c., and finally, excitements of all kinds, far from causing suppression of the menses, do but precipitate the age of puberty, and increase Menstruation. Besides, in warm climates, women are generally endowed with a sanguine-nervous constitution carried to its maximum, and Menstruation is very early, very free, and rarely suppressed. The earliest period for Menstruation, either in India or England, may be taken at 9 years, although ROBERTON, of Manchester, had one case at 8 years, and cites cases occurring at Calcutta, at the same age.* The percentage of cases of Menstruation at Calcutta, under 11 years of age, is 10 per cent.; for England, about 3 per cent. In Venezuela, first Menstruation sets in, in a few very rare cases, at 10 years of age; while only about 10 per cent. occur as early as 11 or 12 years. Hindoo women reach puberty nearly two years earlier than in Europe, a far greater proportion menstruating at 12, 13 and 14 years of age, than in England, where it has not been found that so large a proportion of cases cluster around any particular age, but are scattered more equally over the 12th, 13th, 14th, 15th, 16th, 17th, and even 18th years. PAUL DUBOIS had a case of precocious Menstruation setting in at 9½ years of age, and he places great stress on hereditary influence in bringing about early or late Menstruation. He also had two cases in Paris, in which Menstruation occurred in one at 11 years, the other at 12, and both girls were confined with their first child, one at 13, the other at 14½ years of age; and thinks these cases of premature pregnancy and confinement, with precocious development of the rest of the body, are by no means rare. Menstruation sets in considerably earlier in cities than in the country. It also occurs in the daughters of the rich, in those who have every comfort and luxury, everything which enervates and relaxes, and at the same time excites, at least 9 months before it does in those of the working classes placed in the most comfortable circumstances; and full 14 months, on the average, before it appears in the poorest classes.

* The number of cases of early Menstruation in temperate climates, and even in hot climates, is much smaller than is generally supposed, while the proportion of late cases is much larger in all climates. By reference to the second table, it will be seen that, even in hot climates, as many commence Menstruation as late as 19 years of age, as at 9 years; more at 18 years than at 11; as many at 16 and 17 years, as at 12. While, in temperate climates, more commence to menstruate as late as 23, than as early as 9 years; more at 21 years than at 10; nearly as many at 20 as at 11; full as many at 19 as at 12; more at 18 than at 13; more at 16 than at 14.

WHITEHEAD, thinks especial attention is required in the scrofulous; for although Menstruation is apt to set in too early in them, yet in 226 cases the average time of first Menstruation was between 15 and 16 years of age; still, signs of puberty had commenced earlier than usual, but was slow in being fully accomplished, while regularity as to time and quantity was sustained with difficulty, so that 86 out of the 226 cases, or 38 per cent., required medical treatment, an average far above the general one, which is from 18 to 22 per cent. BENNETT found that only 2 cases out of 5, who menstruated as early as 10 years, did so regularly and easily; only 7 out of 16, who commenced at 11 years; only 8 out of 28, who began at 12 years; 14 out of 35, at 13; 14 out of 42, at 14; also 14 out of 42, at 15; while as many as 20 out of 28, at 16, had, and continued to have their menses regularly, and easily.

TILT has observed, that those who attain to the age of puberty very early, seldom become perfectly regular before the age of 18.

Finally, we may refer to some very curious cases of precocious Menstruation. In one well-established case, Menstruation set in, in an infant, a few days after birth, and continued to recur at the regular periods; in one case, equally well authenticated, the periodical discharge commenced at 9 months of age; in another, at 3 years; in one instance, at 5 years; in another, at 7 years; in 3 cases, at 8 years; and in 11 cases, at 9 years.

TREATMENT.—TILT advances it as a general and judicious rule, that the period of puberty should be delayed as much as possible, at least to the 14th or 16th year, if practicable. Among the remedies most homœopathic to precocious Menstruation, may be mentioned Phosphorus, Ferrum, Phos. ferri, Aloes, Cantharides, Stramonium, and Sabina. The frequent use of hot baths, especially with the addition of mustard; the indulgence in the use of hot, spiced, and stimulating food, and drinks; residence in warm climates, or over-heated houses, or rooms; novel reading, excessive dancing, etc., all tend to produce precocious, frequent, or copious Menstruation. The most antipathic remedies are Conium, Baryta, Secale, and Plumbum, especially if aided by the frequent use of cold baths, scanty clothing, frequent exposure to cold, residence in cold climates, houses, or rooms, bland diet, abstinence from hot tea, and coffee, etc.

Dose.—The most homœopathic remedies, viz., Phosphor., Ferrum, Phos. ferri, Aloe, Cantharides, Stramonium, and Sabina, should be used in comparatively small doses, viz., 1 or 2 grains per dose, of the 1st, 2d, 3d, or 6th trituration of Ferrum acet., or of Phos. ferri; or 1 or 2 drops per dose, of the 1st, 2d, 3d, or 6th dilution of Phosphor., Aloe, Cantharides, Sabina, or of Stramonium, may be given once or twice a day during the interval, or every 2, 4, or 6 hours during the flow. Or, from 2 to 5 granules of the most appropriate of these remedies may be given as often as above directed.

In cases in which these remedies fail to afford relief, larger doses of the strictly antipathic remedies, viz., of Baryta, Conium, Plumbum, and Secale, may be tried; but none but a physician should presume to undertake the responsibility of their administration.

FREQUENT MENSTRUATION.

In 1,045 cases, Whitehead met with 96 women who had returns of Menstruation every 3 weeks regularly, and 134 other cases, in which it returned every 14 days. We have already seen that Roberton supposes, that no less than 28 per cent. of all women have a natural term of only 3 weeks, while in a much smaller class the menses return regularly and normally every fortnight, the free interval being only 9 or 10 days. Condie assumes that in about 18 per cent. the menses return at intervals of very nearly 21 days; that in about 5 per cent. they return every two weeks. In 359 other cases, Whitehead found 36 who were regularly unwell at intervals varying from 20 to 27 days; but whatever the interval, whether 20, 25, or more days, it had always been the same in the same person; in 38 other cases out of 161, the menses recurred every lunar month generally, but set in every 3d or 4th term, from 4 to 7 days earlier, and these deviations were so marked and constant in most instances, as to be expected and anticipated by preparations for these particular times; in 15 other cases out of 161, the menses set in every three weeks generally, but every 3d or 4th return happened from 4 to 7 days later than ordinary; in 14 cases, the interval was 24 days, but occasionally 28 days. In two cases, the returns happened every 18 days; one of these patients, however, had a free interval of a month every 3d, or 4th period; one case menstruated every 28 days as a rule, but at the middle of every third interval, she had an intercurrent discharge, lasting from 30 to 40 hours; two cases menstruated every 14 days, and in one of these the discharge lasted 7 days, leaving a free interval of only 7 days each term. TILT calculates that nearly 17 per cent. of all women have a regular interval of only 3 weeks.

It will be seen that ROBERTON and CONDIE insist that these frequent returns are natural and salutary for some persons. TILT, on the contrary, assumes that the function should be performed neither more nor less frequently than once a month. He says, some physiologists and medical writers have inculcated that it might, with equal benefit to the health, occur every 2, 3, or 4 weeks, and that in fact, all these different types equally fulfil nature's views. But this he believes to be incorrect. His practice has shown that the monthly is the only type of its regular performance, and that any deviation from this rule rarely coincides with good health; most of the cases which have deviated from this law, he says, may be traced to an organic, or merely to a nervous derangement of the ovaries, or of the womb; so much so, that when these diseases are cured, the menstrual function resumes its most habitual type. In one-half of the three-weekly cases which fell under his observation, this frequent recurrencc was explained by the presence of ovario-uterine disease of an organic nature, or of chlorosis; in one case which assumed the fortnightly type, the patient's health was habitually bad. TILT also says, that the fortnightly, or three-weekly appearance depends sometimes merely on a disturbance of that nervous force which must preside over this function, as is evident from the fact, that in many cases in which the irregularity could not be explained by the presence of organic ovario-uterine disease, he had been able to restore the function to its normal type by the use of Sulphate of Quinine. A strong reason which should induce women to desire that this function should be brought to its monthly type, is the additional amount of freedom from infirmity which they acquire, affording them time, taken from suffering, which might be devoted to the cultivation of talents, and the acquirement of happiness. Thus, supposing 4 days of every month to be necessarily given to the performance of this function, then 52 days of inconvenience will have to be endured; but if Menstruation occur every three weeks, there will be 78 days of suffering; or if every fortnight, there will be no less than 104 days thus occupied.—TILT.

TREATMENT.—Nux, Sabina, Aconite, Merc. sol., the Magnet, Platina, and Bryonia, have been decided to be homœopathic when the menses tend to return again almost immediately: viz., Nux, when the menses, which have ceased for one day, return again for some hours. Sabina, when a profuse menstrual flow is apt to set in about three days after the menses have ceased, attended with severe labor-like pains, the blood being partly thin and fluid, partly coagulated, the urine being scanty and red, with strangury, and a leucorrhœal discharge. Aconite, when the menses cease for a day, and then come on again suddenly, and profusely. Mercurius sol., when the menses appear again at the end of 6 days. Application of the Magnet was followed on the next day by the reappearance of the menses, which had ceased for some days, and continued to flow for 10 days more; in another instance, the menses, which had ceased to flow for 10 days, came on again the next day after the application of the Magnet, but only continued for the usual time. The use of Platina was followed on the same day by Menstruation, which was 6 days too soon, and instead of continuing only 3 days, as usual, it persisted for 8 days, attended with a drawing and very unusual pain in the abdomen. The use of Bryonia is said to be followed at times by the reappearance of the menses in the course of a few hours, as much as 8, 14, or even 21 days

days before their regular time. The use of Platina is said to have been followed on the second day of Menstruation, in a case in which there was usually no pain, and the flow was generally quite scanty, by a violent pressure upon the womb, and incessant discharge, attended with griping in the abdomen, and bearing-down pain in the groins.

When Menstruation occurs every 3 weeks, Bryonia, Moschus, Cocculus, Pulsat., Sanguinaria canadensis, and Benzoic acid, are regarded as the most homœopathic remedies. Bryonia is indicated when the menses set in 8 or 14, or 21 days before their time. Moschus when they come on six days too soon and are very profuse—merely smelling of this drug is said to have brough ton Menstruation. Cocculus when it sets in 7 days too soon, attended with distension of the abdomen, and cutting, contractive pains in the bowels from every movement or respiration, and with spasmodic constriction in the rectum; also when it occurs 8 days too early, attended with distension of the abdomen, and a pain in the epigastric region, not only from every movement and step, but also while sitting, with the feeling as if a sharp stone were pressed into the hypogastric region, with soreness to touch. Pusaltilla is said to be indicated in some rare cases, when the menses appear 7 days too soon. Benzoic acid, when the menses occur 8 days too soon and are more copious than usual, but last only 5 days instead of 6 or 7, the discharge being thick and clotted. Sanguinaria, when they set in a week too soon, the discharge being more black than natural.

When Menstruation occurs every 14 days, Ipecac., Bryonia, Nux vom., Nux juglans, Hyosc., Ledum, Prunus spinosa, and Platina, are regarded as the principal remedies. Ipecac. is merely said to be indicated when the menses are renewed every 14 days. Bryonia, when they appear 14 days before their time. Nux vomica, when they reappear on the 14th day again, also Hyosc., Ledum and Prunus spinosa. Nux juglans, when they set in at the end of a fortnight, with pressing and drawing pains in the uterus, and abundant loss of blackish coagulæ. Platina, when the menses, which usually come on every 3 weeks, very moderately, reappear at the end of 14 days, and are very profuse.

According to HEMPEL's Complete Repertory, Sulphuric acid is indicated when the menses occur too soon, and are too profuse. Sulphur, under the same circumstances, especially when they are preceded by chilliness. Oleum animale, in premature Menstruation, attended with pinching pains and colic. Nux vomica, when abdominal spasms are present. Kali carb., in premature Menstruation, when accompanied with debility and drowsiness. Kali bichrom., when premature Menstruation is attended with vertigo, nausea, feverishness, and headache. Graphites, when it occurs too frequently, and is too thin. Asarum, when it happens too soon, and is long continued. Cantharides, when it recurs too frequently, and is profuse and black. Niccolum, when colic and pain in the small of the back are present. Kreosote, when frequent Menstruation is succeeded by a discharge of acrid and bad smelling ichor, causing corrosive itching and smarting of the parts. Laurocerasus, when menses set in too soon, with a profuse and painful discharge of fluid blood, and nocturnal tearing pains in the top of the head. Borax, when there is premature Menstruation, with colic, nausea, and pain extending from the stomach, to the small of the back.

Dose.—1 cr 2 drop doses of the 1st, 2d, 3d, or 6th dilution of Aconite, or of Bryonia, or Cantharides, Cocculus, Hyosc., Ipec., Kreosote, Laurocerasus, Ledum, Nux juglans, Nux vomica, Prunus spinosa, Pulsat., Sabina, Sanguinaria, or of Sulphuric acid, may be given once or twice a day during the interval, and every 2, 4, or 6 hours during the flow, according to the severity of the symptoms. The lower dilutions, and stronger doses of Aconite, Bryonia, Cocculus, Ipecac., Kreosote, and of Sulphuric acid, may be given, than of the other remedies, as some of these are rather styptic and antipathic in their action.

The 1st, 2d, 3d, or 6th trituration of Benzoic acid, Borax, Graphites, Kali bichrom., Kali carb., Merc. sol., Niccolum, Oleum animale, Platina, or of Sulphur, may be used at the same intervals of time as above directed. Or, from 2 to 5 granules may be given per dose, of the remedy most indicated among those just mentioned, and repeated at the same intervals of time.

PROFUSE MENSTRUATION, AND MENORRHAGIA.

Ashwell, in 1,149 cases of uterine disease, met with 79 examples of profuse Menstruation; Madden, in 181 cases, had 43 in which the menses were too copious, and 7 with too prolonged a flow.

Formerly, great stress was placed upon the supposed difference between profuse Menstruation and uterine hæmorrhage. Even Loomis says: "So long as the discharge contains nothing but menstrual fluid, however profuse it may be, it is still Menstruation, and is the most simple unnatural deviation. If, however, the discharge be mixed with blood, we have a more severe form of disease. And if the discharge be pure blood, unmixed with the catamenial secretion, we have a still higher grade." If Whitehead's experiments be reliable, and there is every reason to suppose that they are so, then there is no absolute difference between profuse Menstruation and uterine hæmorrhage. (See p. 20.)

Quite a number of varieties of profuse Menstruation have been described by various authors; the spasmodic and congestive forms, however, have generally been considered the most important. Latterly, the disease has been considered, by one class of physicians, as entirely dependent upon previous derangement of the ovaries; by another class, as always the consequence of inflammation and ulceration of the neck of the womb. Ashwell places great stress upon the presence of a soft and flabby condition of the vagina and uterus, with leucorrhœa, the mouth of the womb being slightly more patulous than usual, but without tenderness or induration. In long-continued menorrhagia, especially in females over 30 or 40 years of age, the presence of a polypus, or malignant disease of the neck of the womb, should always be suspected and examined for.

According to Ashwell, young females are less liable to the disease than those more advanced in life; still, Tilt found first Menstruation to begin with a considerable flow in 30 per cent.; while in 8 per cent. it was said to have amounted to a flooding, and lasted from 8 to 10 days. The plethoric and robust are less frequently subjected to these profuse discharges than females of delicate, susceptible, and feeble constitutions; still, ASHWELL places some stress upon derangement of the liver, coupled with a costive and loaded condition of the bowels, consequent upon luxurious living, and inattention to the state of the bowels.

I consider it entirely unnecessary to give a dull detail of the well-known symptoms which accompany profuse Menstruation in general, but will content myself with succinctly describing the most important pathological varieties of the disorder.

1. *Ovarian Variety.*

As ovarian ovulation is almost always synchronous with Menstruation, it is to be supposed that menorrhagia will be the most common attendant of congestion or inflammation of the ovaries, especially in irritable and nervous women; these are said to form the most obstinate and tedious cases. It is also assumed that there can be no doubt that copious menstrual losses, with double or inter-menstrual periods, are a frequent result of ovarian irritation and congestion; profuse Menstruation is the most common result of these disorders; painful Menstruation is the next in frequency; while the amenorrhœal type is a rare affection. CLARUS has even described a hæmorrhagic variety of ovaritis. In simple and nervous ovaritis, besides the pains about the affected ovary, there are remarkable nervous symptoms, which often mislead the physician to think that he has to deal with hysteria only. But in the hæmorrhagic variety, the nervous symptoms are slight, while the vascular are prominent; the pain and burning in the ovary are also more violent; there is drawing pain along the round ligaments, and at times even the labium of the affected side swells; there is also hæmorrhage from the uterus, which sets in every 8, or 10, or 14 days, with excessive violence, and rapidly leads to anæmia and exhaustion, so that the extremities are apt to become cold, the face pale, and the pulse small, weak, and trembling.

2. *Ulcerative Variety.*

BENNETT says that profuse, prolonged, and too frequent Menstruation, is universally considered to be solely the result of an active or passive state of congestion of the uterus; that is, when it is not occasioned by malignant disease, or by the presence of polypi, or uterine tumors.

This, the general opinion of both ancient and modern pathologists, is founded on ignorance; in reality, in the absence of malignant disease, polypi, or uterine tumors, the quantity of blood lost during Menstruation is seldom permanently increased so as to constitute hæmorrhage, and the menstrual periods are seldom materially prolonged and frequent, unless some chronic, inflammatory, or ulcerative disease of the neck of the womb exist, provided Menstruation be not finally disappearing. BENNETT asserts roundly, that this assumption, on his part, is not the result of theory, but of scrupulous observation, and must become equally evident to all practitioners who will accurately investigate the uterine organs of patients so affected. Congestion of the womb exists, it is true, in menorrhagia, but it is nearly always the result of inflammation of the neck of the womb, and assumes an active or passive character, according to the natural constitution of the patient, and to the amount of reaction produced by the disease on the system at large. If the inflammation of the neck of the womb be of an active nature, and has not had time through its consequences to debilitate the patient, the bleeding will be considered active, or sthenic; if, on the other hand, the disease of the neck has existed for a long time, and caused debility and bloodlessness, then the hæmorrhage will be pronounced asthenic.—BENNETT.

Profuse hæmorrhagic Menstruation may occasionally occur, however, from mere congestion of the uterus, apart from inflammatory disease, as is occasionally seen when Menstruation is ceasing. At the same time, it must be understood that these remarks about the dependence of profuse Menstruation upon ulceration of the neck of the womb, do not apply to females with whom profuse Menstruation is a natural condition, or to those who experience a hæmorrhagic show on particular occasions, as after mental emotions, violent exertion, or some other accidental, and temporary cause.

At the change of life, however, when Menstruation is about to cease definitely, and naturally becomes irregular, profuse menstruation, amounting to flooding, is not uncommon from congestion only, without the presence of any local inflammatory, or ulcerative disease. At this period the menses are apt to disappear for two or more months, and then return again with excessive abundance. It is very seldom, however, even at this period of life, that hæmorrhagic menstrual fluxes occur repeatedly, in the absence of polypi, tumors, or malignant disease, unless there be inflammatory ulceration of the neck of the womb. In nearly all the instances of very obstinate flowing at the change of life, which BENNETT meets with, he finds on examination, that the congestion and hæmorrhage are kept up by inflammatory ulcerative disease. Some of the very worst instances of protracted hæmorrhage that he has ever seen, have been cases of this description. What satisfactorily proves to his mind that the inflammatory ulceration is the cause of the continued hæmorrhage is, that as soon as it is cured, the hæmorrhage ceases.

According to BENNETT, inflammatory ulceration of the neck of the womb is also a common cause of hæmorrhage during pregnancy, and this fact offers an easy and natural explanation of the presumed Menstruation of pregnant females. In those pregnant females for whom he has been consulted, owing to the presence of this phenomenon, he has, on examination, nearly always found, that the blood escaped from an ulceration of the neck of the womb; such ulcerations being peculiarly turgid and luxuriant during pregnancy.

3. *Climacteric Variety.*

ASHWELL thinks that enough attention has not been paid to this form, although it differs so much from the others, that it is a matter of surprise to him that its peculiarities should have been only slightly noticed. He says, it often continues long, occasionally for several years, and frequently in alarming excess. It is often preceded and followed by large, watery, and leucorrhœal discharges, and pain in the uterine and lumbar regions is a common accompaniment. Its sympathetic effects on the brain, lungs, and heart, are occasionally severe, and when the disease has continued long, there is generally coldness of the hands and feet, a feeble and quick pulse, and an anxious, pallid, and sunken countenance. The malady is not confined to one class of women; the plethoric are not more prone to it than the debilitated, and irritable; it rarely or never occurs before 38 or 40 years of age, and sometimes sets in again after Menstruation has been supposed to have ceased.

In mild cases, the symptoms already described terminate after a more or less protracted continuance in the entire cessation of Menstruation; in other and more obstinate examples the symptoms are so extreme as to excite real apprehension. The recurrence of the bleedings is uncertain, although, in general, a catamenial period will be partially observed; occasionally the flow continues for many weeks or months, without any complete cessation, the only appreciable change consisting in a diminished flow; or the discharge may become either watery, or leucorrhœal, or perhaps slightly, or offensively odorous. In many cases there will, at the expiration of a fortnight, or mid-way in the interval between regular monthly periods, be a peculiar, acute, bearing-down pain in the lower part of the uterus, which many patients correctly learn to regard as indicative of a repetition of the menorrhagia. ASHWELL had met with more than several instances, where such hæmorrhages, alarming in degree, have continued for 12, 18, 24, or 48 months, and have ultimately ceased, good health being restored.

In the majority of cases, some enlargement of the uterus, fulness of the neck, and openness of the os, constitute the whole of the diseased change in the womb.

The only other varieties generally admitted are: 1st. The acute, or active menorrhagia, occurring in the plethoric and robust; 2d. The passive, or chronic form, occurring in delicate, hysterical, and exhausted females. A variety characterized by the discharge of what is supposed to be blood and coagulæ, in contradistinction to menstrual secretion, has already been alluded to; there is in reality more difference in quantity, than quality.

Treatment.—It is very important that all cases of profuse Menstruation, or menorrhagia, should be subjected to careful hygienic, or medical treatment. The patient may do much for herself, without consulting a physician, if she will but spare herself as much as possible for a few days before and during the flow; but moderate exercise, and little labor, especially lifting, should be permitted; warm drinks, even of black tea, should be avoided; cold water, or cold, and even iced tea should be taken; injections of cool or cold water into the bowels may be used with benefit, especially if the bowels be costive; tepid, or cool vaginal injections, will often relieve the congestion of the womb, without risk of suppressing the discharge too suddenly. In more severe cases, the recumbent posture, with light clothing, are imperatively required.

ACONITE

Is recommended in cases in which there is arterial excitement, or great irritability; Churchill says that M. West de Soult has published some facts in favor of Aconite as an emmenagogue. Loomis says, it is indicated when there is simply an increased flow of the natural discharge, or if there be nothing but blood passed at the menstrual period, especially if the patient has a yellowish viscous leucorrhœa during the interval, attended with a general feverish condition.

Dose.—As I regard Acon. as antipathic to arterial excitement, 1 or 2 drops of the tincture, or of the 1st, 2d, or 3d decimal dilution, may be given every 2, 4, or 6 hours.

AURUM

Is recommended by Loomis, if the system has been abused by Mercury, or if there be a syphilitic taint, and especially if the neck of the womb be indurated. It perhaps would be no less suitable to that very much larger class of cases in which there is a soft and flabby condition of the vagina and uterus, with leucorrhœa, the mouth of the womb being slightly more patulous than usual. CARRON DE VILLARDS used the Cyanuret of Gold successfully in amenorrhœa, commencing before the expected menstrual period; he solved 3 grains in 8 ounces of alcoholized water, and gave a teaspoonful twice a day, gradually increasing the dose. The metallic gold produces a feeling as if the menses would set in, with labor-like pains in the abdomen; the muriate facilitates the flow of the menses, and causes an earlier occurrence, more profuse flow, and longer continuance of them. VOGT says, if given just before, or soon after Menstruation, it is very apt to cause uterine hæmorrhage. RIECKE says, that it acts powerfully upon the hæmorrhoidal and menstrual flows, while FUNARI, LEGRAND, SOUCHIER, and others, have used it allopathically in amenorrhœa. If given in full doses, it is apt to induce persistent heat in the stomach, increase of appetite, full, strong pulse, general excitement of the nervous system, sleeplessness, restlessness in the legs, loquacity, redness of the face, starting up from sleep, vertigo, increased flow of offensive, thick, and sedimentous urine, or else an abundant discharge of clear and beautiful amber-colored water, with increased warmth in the vulva, congestion to the pelvis, excitement of the genital organs, dry tenesmus, and increased warmth and moisture of the skin.

Dose.—NOACK advises 1 or 2 grains, per dose, of the 1st, 2d, or 3d triturations, dry upon the tongue, every 3d night during the 1st week of the interval; every 2d night during the 2d week; every night during the 3d week, and from 1 to 4 times a day during the flow. Or, 2 or 3 globules may be given as often.

ALOE.

This is one of the most homœopathic remedies to menorrhagia, especially when connected with portal congestion and hæmorrhoids. BRAITHWAITE says, that it acts upon the portal system may fairly be deduced from the very peculiar state into which the hæmorrhoidal vessels are thrown by the congestions which so rapidly occur after a dose of this drug has been taken, and also by the condition of the uterine vessels, which has led to its employment as an emmenagogue. It is apt to irritate the rectum, giving rise in some instances to hæmorrhoids, and also has a decided tendency to the uterus, for its influence in promoting Menstruation is by no means confined to cases in which its action on the neighboring rectum is most conspicuous.—(Wood & Bache.) Cullen says, that it is apt to excite heat and irritation about the rectum, with tenesmus, and bring on a sanguineous discharge. Pereira asserts, that it causes a determination of blood to the uterus, and fulness of its blood-vessels, especially of its veins, and thus uterine irritation and menorrhagia are apt to be induced, and increased by it. Wedekind and Fothergill say, that it exerts a specific stimulant action on the venous system of the abdomen and pelvis, causes increased secretion of bile, irritation about the rectum, vascular excitement of the sexual organs, piles, strangury, immoderate flow of the menses, racking pains in the loins, and labor-like pains. Sobernheim says, that the congestive power of Aloe may go so far as to cause a flow of blood from the kidneys, uterus, and rectum. Dierbach says, in young persons it readily excites febrile symptoms, with a quick pulse, and troublesome sensation of warmth in the abdomen. Harnisch and Noack say, that it may cause burning when urinating, violent pain in the kidneys, scanty and hot urine, discharge of blood from the urethra, tenesmus, aching, and heaviness in the pelvis, aching and burning in the sacral region, erections and pollutions, excitement of the hæmorrhoidal and uterine vessels, and even a similar action in the whole vascular system, so that the pulse will become fuller and harder, the mouth dry, with throbbing and aching in the region of the liver, and congestion of blood to the head and chest.

Still, Eberle says: Would not Dr. Dewees consider Aloe a very improper allopathic remedy in the menorrhagias of young, sanguineous, and robust females? He no doubt would, and why? Because experience has shown that this drug is among the most efficient agents for exciting the uterine vessels, and directing the afflux of blood to them. Yet this very medicine, given in small doses, but frequent ones, deserves to be accounted the best remedy we possess against those protracted, exhausting, and obstinate hæmorrhages from the uterus, which occur in females of nervous, relaxed, and phlegmatic habits, about the critical period of life."—EBERLE.

Dose.—NOACK recommends 1 or 2 drop doses of the pure tincture, or of the 2d or 3d dilution; or from 3 to 5 granules may be given, every ½, 1, or 2 hours, in severe cases; once or twice a day in sub-acute attacks.

BELLADONNA.

According to LOOMIS, it will be especially indicated if the erect posture, or walking produces a pressure downwards of the internal genital organs, attended with shooting pain, particularly if there is a severe throbbing and pressing pain in the head, with fulness and a sensation of swimming in the brain; or if there be prolapsus or induration of the uterus, dryness of the vagina, and the menses return too frequently, and are made up of clear red blood, and fetid clots. It is very certain, however, that Bellad. does not exert nearly so specific an action upon the uterine organs as Stramonium, although it has been recommended from experience, against profuse and premature appearance of the menses, and in menorrhagia, when accompanied by a painful pressure upon the womb, violent pain in the small of the back, and the discharge is rather dark and coagulated. It has also cured cases of profuse Menstruation brought on by exertion in heavy lifting, when there was violent pain in the whole abdomen, the discharge being so copious that bright red blood flowed continuously in a thin stream, the pulse being full, hard, and frequent. Belladonna causes such violent congestion to the head and upper parts of the body, that it may almost be supposed to exert a derivative effect in congestions to the womb and pelvic organs.

Dose.—It is probable that larger doses of Bellad. are required in affections of the lower part of the body, than in those of the upper. NOACK prefers 1 or 2 drop doses of the 1st, 2d, 3d, 6th, or 12th dilution, repeated every 2, 3, or 4 hours, in sub-acute attacks; every 5, 10, 15, or 30 minutes, in very severe cases. If preferred, from 3 to 6 pellets may be dissolved in a wineglassful of water, and a teaspoonful given as often as above directed; or 2 or 3 granules may be given dry upon the tongue. In BEAUVAIS' Clinique, of 106 cases of profuse Menstruation, only 2 were treated with Bellad.; in both instances the 30th dilution was used, but the cases progressed in severity until the expulsion of large clots from the womb brought relief.

BRYONIA.

We have already seen that this remedy is homœopathic to frequent Menstruation; it has also been found useful in menorrhagia and abdominal sufferings, brought on by a blow upon the abdomen, when there was a continual sanguineous discharge from the vagina, which increased to hæmorrhage every three weeks, attended with burning pains in the stomach, increased by every motion, and becoming intolerable from the least exertion, attended with paroxysms of anguish and chilliness. It was also useful in a case of profuse Menstruation, brought on by the excessive use of herb-teas; after several pounds of blood had been lost, the patient's face being pale and sunken, her strength gone, pulse variable, now hard and irritable, then small and weak; attended with violent burning pain in the small of the back, but commencing at the pit of the stomach; with paroxysmal, violent pressure in the abdomen, nausea, vertigo; discharge of large lumps of dark and coagulated blood without pain, while walking, and even while lying down; no appetite, costiveness, sleeplessness, and frequent chills.

Bryonia is allied to Colchicum in its action, and is homœopathic to profuse Menstruation occurring in rheumatic subjects, and those disposed to rheumatic diarrhœa. KASPAR thinks that Bryonia has no affinity for the sexual organs, except in so far as the serous envelopes are affected; but it is undoubtedly homœopathic to profuse Menstruation from a rheumatic affection of the serous and muscular coats of the uterus.

Dose.—NOACK says, 1 or 2 drops of the pure tincture of Bryonia, or of the 1st, 2d, or 3d dilution, may be given frequently in acute cases; once or twice a day in chronic affections; or 2 or 3 granules may be given dry upon the tongue; or 5 or 6 globules may be solved in a wineglassful of water, and 1 or 2 teaspoonfuls given as often as above directed. In Beauvais' 106 cases, Bryonia was only used 5 times; the 15th dilution in 2 cases, the 18th in 1, and the 30th in 2 cases; in 4 cases it was only given after the discharge had been moderated by Crocus, China, or some other remedy; in the 5th case, it relieved the most violent rheumatic and spasmodic affection of the uterus, attended with profuse discharge of blood.

CARBO ANIMALIS

Cured a case of profuse Menstruation of 16 months' standing, after many other remedies had been used in vain; the discharges recurred at intervals of 8 or 10 days, being fetid and putrid, the patient was also affected with a painful hardness in the region of the liver, and with intense pain around the small of the back, and in the groin.

Dose.—Noack says, that 1 or 2 grains may be given dry upon the tongue, once or twice a day, in chronic attacks; it is rarely used in acute affections. Or from 2 to 4 granules may be given every night and morning.

CHAMOMILLA.

This remedy may be regarded as the "Catnip of Homœopathy." Vogt classes it among the *Excitantia volatilia*, or those remedies which cause a transient arousing of the irritable system. It is supposed to act principally upon those splanchnic nerves which ramify in the cavities of the abdomen and pelvis; still its action is so gentle that it is decreed to be rarely useful in severe and obstinate cases. In old-school practice it has been principally used against nervous pains, especially in colics, hysterical spasms, spasmodic affections of females occurring during Menstruation, or before or after confinement, in spasms of the chest or heart, in hysterical asthma, slight rheumatic pains and colics. It is regarded as important, if Chamomilla be expected to afford relief in these affections, that they should have just commenced, not be very severe, and arise from accumulation of wind in the bowels, or be of a rheumatic or nervous character.

Loomis thinks that it is peculiarly adapted to that excessive sensibility of the nervous system, which precedes and accompanies the flow, in nearly all cases of menorrhagia from irritable uterus. If administered on the first indication of the approach of the menses, either alone or in alternation with Coffea, Nux, or Pulsatilla, it will often mitigate the sufferings very much, although it will do but little towards removing any organic change in the uterus, or ovaries. It is best suited to those cases where the pains are spasmodic and paroxysmal, resembling labor-pains. It is most useful against the sufferings which precede the commencement of the menstrual flow, although if there be excessive irritation of all the sexual organs, with much itching, it may be beneficial during the flow, especially if there be a profuse discharge of mucus with the menses. Leadam thinks Chamomilla is to be preferred when the discharge of blood is dark, blackish, and coagulated, occurring in gushes, with pressure upon the womb like labor-pains, attended with frequent desire to pass water, and drawing or tearing pains in the thighs and legs; with irritability of temper, fainting fits, coldness of the limbs, paleness of the face, and thirst. It has relieved some cases of menorrhagia after parturition, even when the patient was almost unconscious from loss of blood, the face and body being cold and pale, the pulse scarcely perceptible, and the blood flowing violently. Also, cases of metrorrhagic Menstruation, when the blood flowed continuously, intermixed with large, black coagulæ, the whole having a fetid smell; when the pulse was full but not hard, great weakness being present, with roaring in the ears, dimness of sight and heaviness of the head, followed by fainting fits whenever the patient attempted to raise herself; in some of these cases, Nux may be required for constipation, and China must be used to remove the subsequent debility.

Although Cham. and Coffee are said only to relieve slight and recent cases, yet they have cured one very severe case. A woman, aged 32, had suffered for 3 months with metrorrhagia, to such an extent that fainting ensued, and the patient was thought to be dead. On the physician's arrival, he found the tapers already lighted, and a number of ladies engaged in prayer around the bed; her pulse was almost imperceptible, as also the motions of the heart; five or six spoonfuls of black Coffee were introduced successively into the patient's mouth, whereby consciousness was restored in a quarter of an hour. On the following morning, a dose of Chamomilla was given, which stopped the bleeding and completed the cure.—Brit. Jour. Hom., vol. 8, p. 426.

Dose.—In the above cases, the 3d and 4th dilutions were used. It is, however, such a very mild remedy, that several drops of the pure tincture may be given every ½, 1, 2, or more hours; or the same quantities of the 1st, 2d, or 3d dilution may be used for very sensitive persons. In the very rare cases in which these, or still stronger doses do not suffice, the higher dilutions may be tried, 2 or 3 globules to be given dry upon the tongue, as often as above directed. In BEAUVAIS' 106 cases, Cham. was used only 7 times; the Tinct. in 1 case promptly relieved a hæmorrhage of 3 weeks' duration; the 4th dilution was given in 1 case; the 6th in two cases; the 9th in 1; and the 12th in 2 cases, but mostly with equivocal success.

CANTHARIDES.

LOOMIS says that this remedy will prove useful when there is a discharge of black blood, attended with severe pains, especially if there be swelling of the neck of the womb, accompanied with corrosive leucorrhœa both before and after Menstruation, and by burning pain when urinating. There is a great deal of old-school experience in favor of the use of Cantharides in amenorrhœa and scanty Menstruation, but little or none in profuse Menstruation. DEWEES says, when Madder fails in amenorrhœa, he commences in recent cases with Tincture of Cantharides, in doses of 35 or 40 drops, and rarely increases the quantity more than 10 or 15 drops beyond the original dose, as the former *moderate* (!!) doses have always been found sufficient by him when the medicine would succeed at all. PEREIRA says, in consequence of the specific stimulus communicated to the bladder by Cantharides, it has been supposed that the same influence might be extended to the womb, and thus this remedy has been employed as a stimulating emmenagogue; in some cases with apparent benefit, but frequently without any obvious effect. Abortion has occasionally happened from its employment, as Pereira himself witnessed in one case. Wood says, in old cases of menorrhagia, where the uterus is very feeble and relaxed, remedies calculated to stimulate this organ directly have been recommended, such as Aloetic preparations, and even Cantharides and Sabina; but these must be employed with great caution, i. e., in small or homœopathic doses. A writer in Wood's Quarterly Retrospect says, in asthenic menorrhagia, Cantharides is a powerful and efficient medicine, and, combined or alternated with Nux vomica, it is capable of relieving the patient in a short time; he advises the tremendous doses of from 36 to 60 drops of a mixture of equal parts of Tinct. Cantharides and Tinct. Nux vomica, to be given 3 times a day in sugar and water; or the Cantharides may be given alone; and as soon as the flow ceases, Ferrum or China are advised to obviate the consequent debility.

Dose.—Noack recommends 1 or 2 drop doses of the 1st, 2d, 3d, or 6th dilution, repeated once or twice a day in chronic cases, although they may be given every ½, 1, or 2 hours in more urgent attacks. For very susceptible persons, from 1 to 3 granules may be given as often as above directed.

CHINA.

This remedy, according to Leadam, is useful when the discharge is black and clotted, occurring at intervals, with pressure upon the womb, and jerking movements of the body, proceeding from depletion rather than spasm, and attended with painful tension of the abdomen; or when the following symptoms arise in consequence of great loss of blood: sense of weight in the head, vertigo, dulness of sensibility, and drowsiness, the patient being cold and blue; it may also be given after the attack has passed over, or during the intervals between the frequent returns of the menses, as part of the constitutional treatment. It proved useful in one case, in which there was continual dizziness, with headache over the whole head, constant glittering before the eyes, humming in the ears, dryness of the mouth without thirst, pain in the abdomen resembling labor pains, extending from the small of the back to the bladder; desire to urinate, with scanty discharge; scanty and hard stools, with much pressing; unusual debility, sleeplessness, frightful dreams, palpitations of the heart, and anxiety; constant chilliness, with coldness of the hands and feet; forgetfulness and anxiety, with fear of dying; all proceeding from, and attended with continual discharge of blood and clots from the uterus and vagina.

Dose.—The 16th dilution was used in one case. NOACK advises 1, 2, or several drops, per dose, of the pure Tincture; or the same quantities of the 1st, 2d, or 3d dilution, repeated every ½, 1, or 2 hours in severe cases; every 2, 4, or 6 hours in milder attacks. In some cases, from 2 to 5 globules may be given as often. In BEAUVAIS' 106 cases, China was used 17 times, mostly to relieve the subsequent debility after the hæmorrhage had been stopped by other remedies. The 12th dilution was used in 7 cases, relieving the debility about as promptly as if full doses of Bark had been given; the 2d dilution in 1 case; the Tinct. in 2 cases; 6th in 1 case; 15th in 2 cases; 16th in 1 case; 9th in 1 case. In 1 instance only did it exert a marked influence upon the flow, when given in a high dilution.

CALCAREA.

According to LEADAM, it will be found useful when the menses are too profuse, or too frequent in their recurrence, and the patient has a scrofulous diathesis. HAHNEMANN says, that it will never be given with benefit when there is a deficiency of the menstrual flow. It is more beneficial when given during the interval, in order to correct that condition of the uterus and general system upon which the unnatural state of the menstrual function depends; it may be given alone, or in alternation with China, Nux and Sulphur. LOOMIS says, that Calcarea is one of the most important remedies in certain conditions of the uterine organs, when attended by profuse and premature discharge; but it is seldom indicated when there is an irritable uterus. If, however, there be shooting pains about the mouth of the womb, with aching pain in the vagina, and a sensation of bearing down, or if there be a burning pain in the womb, it will be of use to administer a single dose during the interval; he says a *single* dose only, because he has never repeated Calcarea with advantage in cases where the menses returned too soon, or were too profuse, but, on the contrary, a repetition of the dose has invariably made the case worse.

But Dr. Patzack has rendered himself famous by his methodical use of Calcarea, aided by Nux, China, and Sulphur. He says, it is of great importance to give remedies during the period intervening between the catamenial discharges, in consequence of which it is generally unnecessary to act during the flow. Nux vom., China, Sulphur and Calcarea have proved eminently successful in his hands, not only in regulating the menses, but also in removing the bad consequences of a too frequent and too copious hæmorrhage, both in the organs of generation, and in the system generally. He adopts the following methodical use of these remedies: on the evening of the 1st day after the cessation of the menses, he gives a dose of Nux vom.; thirty-six hours afterwards, he administers a dose of China in the morning; in thirty-six hours more, another dose of Nux in the evening, and so on; this alternation of Nux and China, every thirty-six hours, is persisted in during the first half of the intermenstrual period. The treatment of the latter half of the interval is begun with a dose of Sulphur, followed in 2 days after by a dose of Calc. carb., after which these two medicines are continued alternately during the remainder of the latter half of the interval. Patzack says, that the effect of this treatment, even in cases of very long standing, was most surprising to him, viz., a speedy restoration of the general health, and a more regular appearance and duration of the recurring catamenia. It will of course be seen, that he not only does not fear, but practically does not meet with the bad consequences from a repetition of the doses of Calcarea, upon which so much stress is laid by Loomis.

Patzack corroborates his assertions by the recital of several cases:

CASE 1. Baroness C., aged 27, lively and somewhat delicate, had had 5 confinements within 6 years, flowed excessively each time, and had suffered with piles. As she did not nurse her last child, the catamenia appeared soon after parturition, very copiously, and continued to do so whenever she was not pregnant. Ipecac. relieved an attack of flowing; Nux and China improved her strength and relieved the piles; afterwards she took Sulphur and Calcarea in alternation, with such good effect, that the menses were nearly natural at their next appearance, and she was completely cured in a few months.

CASE 2. Baroness R., a sister of the above, also delicate, had lost much blood 6 years before at a confinement, and never since had been able to regain her former strength; her menses had also become not only too copious, but also of too long duration; she had continued pressing, and gnawing pains in the regions of the ovaries, but more particularly on the left side, which were aggravated by any mental or physical excitement, especially just before Menstruation, to such a degree that they spread over the whole abdomen, in the region of the bladder, in the lumbar region, and downwards from the hips, so that it was impossible for her to take any exercise. Sulphur and Calcarea, continued for 3 months, completely restored her, with the exception of the pains in the ovaries, which were finally, and perfectly relieved by Bryonia.

CASE 3. Mrs. A., aged 30, of feeble constitution, had suffered for years with too copious and frequent Menstruation, to which leucorrhœa had been added for the last year; and cardialgia, with pressing pains extending to the back, for the last 5 months. She also had nausea, without actual vomiting, and her bowels were obstinately costive. She was entirely cured in 2 months by the above remedies.

CASE 4. Mrs. Von B., aged 34, had menstruated too copiously ever since the first appearance of the menses, but still more so since her marriage. As a consequence of such excessive loss of fluids, she had an extraordinary degree of sensibility of the nervous system, so that even trifling causes, particularly fright and anger, would produce an unusual degree of excitement in the vascular and nervous systems, such as palpitations, trembling, pain in the stomach, headache, the most violent toothache, &c.; she also had great debility, irritability, and low spirits. She too was cured by the above remedies.

CASE 5. Mrs. W., aged 40, of vigorous constitution and large frame, had miscarried several times, been troubled with too copious and frequent menstrual discharge, great debility, and frequently returning and most violent cardialgia, for the last 15 years. Nux did not benefit her much, but after the first few doses of China, she mended rapidly; Sulphur and Calcarea were then given, and the next Menstruation occurred later, and lasted only 5 days. She recovered perfectly, and did not relapse in 2½ years.

CASE 6. Mrs. F., aged 35, apparently in vigorous health, had suffered with excessive general weakness since the birth of her 5th child; to this was added vertigo, frequently accompanied by violent headache, for which she had been bled repeatedly; besides this, her menses returned very copiously every 3 weeks. She improved much in 4 weeks, and finally recovered completely, under the use of Nux, China, Sulphur, and Calcarea.

Dose.—Five chronic cases were cured by Calc. 30, 2 doses every week; the 3d and 4th dilutions have also effected cures when given every 2 or 8 days, or at longer intervals. NOACK advises 2, or 3 grain doses of the 1st, 2d, or 3d dilution, to be given once or twice a day, or only every 2d, 4th, or 6th day. Or from 3 to 5 globules may be given as often as above directed.

CINNAMON

Is often recommended as homœopathic to hæmorrhage from the uterus, but its action is generally described as aromatic, carminative, and astringent, and hence antipathic to many atonic discharges. DIERBACH says, its continued use is apt to cause costiveness, and that it is supposed to exert a specific action on the uterus, while the Tannin which it contains renders it a proper remedy in the treatment of chronic hæmorrhages and blennorrhœas, especially of the genital organs; it has also been used to increase, and sustain labor-pains, and is thought to be especially useful in chronic uterine hæmorrhages.

Dose.—It would seem to be downright folly to use as small doses of this remedy, as of the Bellad., Arsen., and other powerful remedies, especially in uterine hæmorrhage, to which it is not especially homœopathic. Very powerful and strictly homœopathic remedies may possibly be used with success in infinitesimal doses; but very mild, and non-homœopathic medicines must be used in more massive quantities. The quantities recommended in the old school will probably be the safest, and most effective in profuse Menstruation.

CROCUS.

According to Leadam, it is an excellent remedy when there is an escape of black, lumpy, viscid blood, increased by the least movement, attended with cutting pains deep in the abdomen, extending to the small of the back; one of its most characteristic symptoms is the sensation of something alive in the abdomen, in the form of a ball, most marked when the flowing is most active. It is thought to be suitable in attacks of profuse Menstruation which have arisen from dancing, or taking stimulating drinks during the menstrual period; or when palpitation, anxiety, and melancholy, jerking and creeping in the limbs, thirst, heavy dreams, and starting on going to sleep prevail. It has cured cases of chronic metrorrhagia, when there was an almost constant discharge of dark, tenacious blood, especially early in the morning, intermingled with black coagulæ, and alternating with a flow of thin, bloody water, like flesh water. When there were free intervals of only 3 or 4 days, during which there was a heavy pain in the groins; or when there is almost constant pain in the groin, and drawing in the small of the back; but little appetite, which is quickly satisfied; sensation as if there were something alive in the epigastric region; frequent attacks of anxiety, with flushes of heat over the whole body, and prickling in the skin as if perspiration would break out; when the patient is almost always languid and weary; sleeps but little, has a livid complexion, and sunken cheeks. *Platina* may be required in alternation, if the menses continue to return every

14 days, rather profusely, with colic and labor-like pressing downwards in the pelvis, although Crocus will generally moderate the discharge at each menstrual period.

Crocus also cured a case of menorrhagia caused by fright; the patient had for 19 weeks passed large quantities of dark, fetid, black blood, uninterruptedly, but without pain; around the umbilicus there was a sensation as if a ball were moving to and fro; she also had a beating pain in the left side of the head, especially in the morning, affecting the left eye, the lids of which were inclined to stick together; the loss of blood had already caused dimness of vision, dizziness, fainting fits, complete want of appetite, almost continual nausea, and excessive languor; the limbs felt bruised, and the legs were slightly swollen; the patient was constantly chilly, slept badly, and was costive; her complexion had become sallow, she was emaciated, sad, obstinate, and ill-humored. Ipecac. assisted in removing the discharge of blood. Nux removed the constipation; and Ferrum muriaticum the pains and swelling of the legs.

Crocus also cured a case of menorrhagia occurring every 8 days, at new and full moon, the blood being viscid and blackish. Also another case, from being overheated at the time of Menstruation; the patient already lay as if lifeless, was unable to open her eyes from excessive weakness; her face and lips were pale, and she fainted away when she attempted to move; she had headache, chilliness, discharge of dark and fetid blood from the vagina, without pain; she felt a sensation as if something alive were in the abdomen, was dizzy, anxious, and her pulse was quick and scarcely perceptible; her complexion was anæmic and sallow. China 4, removed the remaining debility.

Of Beauvais' 106 cases, 18 were cured by *Crocus*, viz., 1 case that had lasted more than a year, was cured in 3 months, by the 1st dilution; another, which had continued for 6 months, was relieved in 3 days, by the use of the 1st dilution; a third, of 4 months' duration, was removed in 11 hours, by the 3d dilution; a fourth, of long duration, by the 1st dilution; a fifth, which had continued 19 weeks, was successfully removed in 20 days, by the 3d dilution; 4 other cases of from several to 9 days' duration, were cured in about 1 day, by the Tinct.; a similar case was successfully treated by the 1st dilution; 4 cases, of several days continuance, were cured in from a few hours to 1 day, by the 3d dilution; one case, of several hours' duration, in a few hours, by the 2d dilution; another, by the 4th potency; and one, which had lasted for 2 days, profusely, was cured in 2 days, by the 5th dilution. The higher potencies do not seem to have been used in a single instance.

The celebrated KOPP says, that in his hands, Crocus has produced rapid relief in several cases of menorrhagia; sometimes he used the 1st or 2d dilution, at other the pure tincture; in some instances only a single drop was required in order to diminish steadily, and finally check, a profuse hæmorrhage, without any subsequent bad consequences. Other patients took 2 or 3 small doses of Crocus at intervals of 12 or 24 hours.

CASE 20. A young lady always menstruated so profusely, that she was unable to leave her bed. One drop of Tinct. Crocus generally relieved her in the course of 1 day.—KOPP.

CASE 21. A lady aged 40, was taken suddenly with violent pains in the back and stomach, followed by such a violent hæmorrhage, that her life seemed in danger; the blood was black and often came away in large clots. After 1 dose, of 1 drop Tinct. Crocus, the flow lessened considerably on the same day; on the 2d day, nothing but colored water was discharged; and on the 3d day she was well.—KOPP.

CASE 22. A young lady, aged 16, menstruated with all the violence of a metrorrhagia. She took 1 drop of Crocus, 1st dilution, and a similar dose on the next day; she was cured by the 2d evening.—KOPP.

CASE 23. A lady, aged 42, after using Bryonia 18, Sabina 12, Platina 2, scruple doses of Ferrum carb., and tablespoonful doses of infusion of Sabina, with very partial success, was cured in a few days by Crocus, 1st and 2d dilution. Nux 18 was also given several times, and acted upon the bowels every time it was administered.—Kopp.

CASE 24. A lady, aged 27, from over exertion on the 10th day after her confinement, was attacked with violent uterine hæmorrhage. Two doses of Crocus 1st, relieved her entirely in 24 hours.

CASE 25. A lady, aged 42, whose metrorrhagia, with discharge of black blood and clots, had long resisted antiphlogistic and styptic remedies, was cured by two doses of Crocus.

CASE 26. Sabina is regarded as the best homœopathic remedy, when the flow is of a bright red color; Crocus, when it is dark, black, and colored. A young woman was taken with flowing on the 2d day after confinement; the discharge was said to be bright red in color, and a dose of Sabina 18, was given without benefit. Then 1 dose of Sabina 3, and one of Crocus 3, were sent; the former to be given if the discharge was bright red in color; the latter if the contrary was the case. The discharge was found to be dark and clotted, and the Crocus was consequently given; improvement set in, in the course of half an hour, and a cure was rapidly effected.—Rau.

CASE 27. A lady, aged 36, had suffered with returns of profuse Menstruation for 6 months; the discharge generally lasted about 15 days; 2 doses of Crocus relieved one attack promptly; and a repetition of the same treatment, at the three succeeding monthly periods, cured her entirely.—Duplat.

CASE 28. A lady, in the 4th month of pregnancy, was suddenly seized during the night with pain, attended with flooding to an alarming extent; the blood was of a dark color. Crocus arrested without altogether stopping the discharge; Belladonna restrained it still more, and in less than an hour entirely subdued it. It recurred, however, on the following night to a considerable extent, but was completely stopped by the same remedies. The lady then went her full time, and gave birth to a healthy infant.—Dunsford.

Many other interesting cases are given, but they are too long for insertion here.

It may be well, however, to quote the opinions of various authors about the action of Crocus. Wood and Bache say, that Crocus was formerly considered highly stimulant and anti-spasmodic; in small doses it was supposed to moderately excite different functions, to exhilarate the spirits, relieve pain, and produce sleep; in large doses it may give rise to headache, dizziness, delirium, and stupor. It was also thought to act powerfully upon the uterine system, promoting Menstruation, and on the Continent it is still used as a stimulant, and emmenagogue. Pereira says it was formerly considered to be cordial, aromatic, narcotic, and emmenagogue; Boerhaave regarded it as homœopathic to laughing delirium; Bergius ascribed great mental dejection to its use; Boerhaave and Riverius have declared, that they have seen immoderate uterine hæmorrhage produced by it, which proved fatal in one case. It was at one time esteemed as an anti-spasmodic in asthma, hysteria, and cramp in the stomach, and was used as an emmenagogue, and to promote uterine contraction and the lochial discharge; lastly, it has been employed as a stimulant to the nervous system in hypochondriasis. Neligan says that Crocus is a stimulant of weak power, exerting a specific influence, by no means well marked, over the uterine organs, whence it is generally said to be emmenagogue; on the Continent it bears a high character as a remedy for the severe lumbar pains, which so frequently precede or accompany Menstruation. Sobernheim places it among the pure narcotics, and says that experience has proven it an excellent analeptic remedy for young children, being slightly stimulating, while it also relieves pain and spasm, and hence is often much to be preferred to Opium. It also stands in a specific relation to the female sexual organs, being apt to excite a congestive state of the uterine system, while it also exerts a stimulating, resolving, and fluidizing influence upon the portal system, which is so intimately connected with the menstrual function; hence it facilitates the periodical excretion from the uterus, and has obtained a reputation as a forcing and emmenagogue remedy. It is also supposed to exert a specific curative action upon congestive and spasmodic affections of the chest, especially in those arising from irregularity of the menstrual function. It is decreed to be a main remedy in suppression of the menstrual and lochial secretions, especially when arising from debility and irritability of the uterine system, and attended with pain and spasms. The more plethoric the patient is, the more careful the physician must be in the use of Crocus; but it will afford excellent service when there is torpor of the vascular system in general, and of the uterus in particular, occurring in females of a sluggish and relaxed habit, more or less leucophlegmatic, and predisposed to mucous discharges, and irregularities of Menstruation; it is most useful when the menses are suppressed, entirely absent, irregular, or scanty and difficult. VOGT thinks that it resembles Bellad. in its action more than Opium; that it acts primarily upon the nerves, and next upon the muscular system, being inclined to cause commotions and congestions of blood, and excessive hæmorrhages; it may promote the flow of the menses, and the secretions from the skin, mucous membranes of the air tubes and genital organs, of the kidneys and serous membranes. VOGT also recommends it in nervous and spasmodic affections of the chest and head, when coupled with irregular Menstruation; in disorders of the portal systems, in suppression or scantiness of Menstruation or lochiæ, in weak and irregular contractions of the uterus during confinement. DIERBACH recommends it as a very powerful sedative, pain- and spasm-relieving medicine, especially for young children, in whom it should be used more frequently than Opium; as an anti-spasmodic against hysteria and hypochondria, in spasmodic colic, and spasmodic affections of the chest; also in the spasmodic derangement of Menstruation, against scanty menses, and lochiæ, and against insufficient labor-pains.

Dose.—The majority of cases were cured by the 1st dilution; the 3d dilution, repeated several times a day, has also been found serviceable. NOACK recommends drop doses of the pure tincture, or of the 1st, or 2d dilution, every ½, 1, 2, or 3 hours. STAPF prefers the trituration;—or from 3 to 5 globules may be given per dose.

HYOSCIAMUS.

LEADAM thinks that one of the primary effects of this drug is uterine hæmorrhage, but it is far less homœopathic to this disorder than Stramonium. It is said to be indicated when the menses are profuse, and attended with delirium, the blood being of a bright red; or by spasms, interrupted by jerks or startings of single limbs, followed by rigidity of the joints; or being preceded by hysteric pains, or hysterical laughter, and attended with spasmodic pains and trembling of the hands and feet, or by difficult micturition with pressing, or fainting fits with convulsive movements; or restlessness, the body being hot, with swelling of the veins, full and quick pulse, dulness of the senses, obscuration of the sight and delirium.

Dose.—NOACK prefers 1 or 2 drop doses of the 1st, 2d, 3d, or 6th dilution, to be given at short intervals in severe cases, or only once a day in milder attacks. Or from 3 to 5 globules may be given per dose, every ¼, ½, or 1 hour, in severe cases; every 4, 6, or 8 hours, in less urgent attacks.

FERRUM

Is said by LEADAM to be applicable as a homœopathic remedy when the blood is at times fluid, at others black and clotted, its discharge being attended with labor-pains in the abdomen and groins, great vascular excitement, heat and redness of the face, fulness and hardness of the pulse. *China* is homœopathic to an almost similar state.

According to RÜCKERT, it has cured metrorrhagia occurring after parturition, with all the above symptoms, and frequent chills, headache, and vertigo, constipation, and hot urine; also cases of profuse Menstruation, amounting to hæmorrhage, and when there was violent erethism of the vascular system.

In old school practice, Iron is recommended in all passive hæmorrhages. WOOD advises it in cases where the system and uterus are both relaxed, and the bleeding appears to be sustained by this condition. As the coagulability of the blood depends mainly upon the quantity and quality of it contained fibrin, and Ferrum is well known to diminish the quantity of fibrin in the blood, it is a matter of course that it will tend to produce hæmorrhage, if it be given too long, or in too large doses. The Nitrate of Silver exerts, perhaps, the most powerful action of any known remedy, upon the coagulability of the fibrin, and has been used very successfully against obstinate metrorrhagia.

Dr. Liedbeck says he has used Iron in the same doses as recommended by Rademacher in severe hæmorrhages of the womb, viz., 30 drops per dose, of the Liquor ferri mur. oxyd. Ph. Bor., in 8 ounces of distilled water, with the addition of two drachms of Gum Arabic. Even hæmorrhages from cancer have diminished more than from any other remedy. The loss of blood from any cause whatever, even from excoriations and ulcerations of the os uteri and vagina, has either diminished, or the patient has at least felt stronger and livelier. He has also obtained a perfect cure in some cases, where there were no indications for the use of Sabina, or Crocus, which, generally, as well as Belladonna, China, and Secale, have been his best remedies.

CASE.—Mrs. B., aged about 40, had always had profuse Menstruation; since her last confinement, 4 years ago, she has suffered from almost constant hæmorrhage from the womb, escaping only about 8 days in every month; she had a great deal of inflammation of the womb, accompanied with pains and tenderness of the abdomen; she had been repeatedly purged, was much weakened, and easily provoked to tears; the blood was dark, like cherry jelly; the neck of the uterus was swollen; she was tender in coitus; had a soreness of the chest, and a feeling of anxiety, with great difficulty in ascending a hill, or walking up stairs.

Treatment and Result.—One tablespoonful of the above mentioned Iron mixture was given every hour; she felt sleepy after the medicine, had a light pain in the stomach, and some dark and loose evacuations from the bowels, but still she felt better, and the bleeding diminished; there was, however, soreness about the os coccygis, and some pain and difficulty in sitting. The uterus was tilted towards the right, and the right leg was swelled. The bleeding subsided entirely on the fourth day of the treatment. Ten days after, the patient had gained in flesh and appearance, and felt quite like another person; there had been no return of the bleeding. LIEDBECK exclaims: Could these results have been obtained by high dilutions of Iron, or of any other remedy? He believes not, and thinks that those who use the high dilutions, would do well to publish some of their cases.

Dose.—NOACK prefers 1 or more drops per dose, of the pure tincture, or of the 1st dilution, repeated once or twice a day, in chronic cases; every 2, 3, or 4 hours, in more urgent attacks. Or ½ or 1 grain doses of the 1st or 2d trituration, may be given. In very susceptible persons, 2 or 3 granules may be administered as often as above directed. Of BEAUVAIS' 106 cases, Ferrum was used in 5, viz.: in one case, in the 3d dilution, to remove swelling of the feet, after the cure of the menorrhagia by Crocus, Ipec., and Nux; in a 2d case, a strong, plethoric woman with hæmorrhage, on the 13th day after confinement, was quickly relieved of pain and hæmorrhage, by 2 drops Tinct. Iron, in 4 ounces of water, given in divided doses; a case of long standing, was cured in 2 days, by Ferrum metallicum; a case of 9 days duration, was increased for 2 hours under the use of Ferrum, 6th dilution, but in 10 hours more the flow was reduced more than one-half, and ceased entirely on the next day.

IGNATIA

Is recommended when the menses come away in masses of coagulated blood, with crampy pains in the womb, like labor pains, and with a tendency to spasms. This remedy, like Nux, acts most specifically upon the muscular fibres of the uterus and the motor nerves, and hence is most homœopathic to spasmodic menorrhagia.

Dose.—Ignatia is a powerful remedy, of which 1 or 2 drops may be given of the 2d, 3d, or 6th dilution, every 1, 2, or 4 hours in some attacks; or once, or twice a day, or only every 2, 5, or more days, in chronic cases. In exceptional cases, from 1 to 3 globules may be given as often as above recommended. In BEAUVAIS' 106 cases, Ignatia was used only twice, viz., in 1 case in the 6th dilution, in the other in the 18th. In both cases the flowing had already ceased before the Ignatia was given to remove spasmodic, dyspeptic, or hæmorrhoidal affections.

IPECAC.

Leadam says that it is recommended when there is much weakness, and the bleeding is of a passive character, attended with cutting pains about the navel, pressing down towards the uterus and anus, coldness, shivering, paleness of the face, and heat within the head, the discharge being of a bright red.

According to Rückert, Ipec. 1st, one drop per dose, cured a case of metrorrhagia in the course of a couple of hours, which had been treated unsuccessfully for 9 months. Also a case of metrorrhagia in a pregnant female; from over exertion, she was seized with nausea, a feeling of warmth in the abdomen, and slight dizziness, followed by flow of blood from the uterus, pain in the small of the back, weakness and heaviness of the legs, and weariness of the body.

Ashwell recommends Ipecac. in spasmodic menorrhagia, and gives an illustrative case: A widow, aged 37, of spare habit, but not weak, had been menorrhagic for several years, and suffered habitually from dyspepsia. Menstruation had lasted only 2 days, but for the last 24 hours the parxoysms of pain and spasm about the womb had been very severe; much blood had been lost by gushes, and many large clots had been expelled; the spasms still continued; the pulse was quick (130) and irritable, but neither full nor hard; she was chilly and faint; her face pallid and anxious; and she had had no sleep from the commencement of the attack, although there had been long intervals of freedom from pain. At the commencement of the disease, three years since, she had been bled and purged with decidedly injurious effects.

Treatment.—One scruple of powdered Ipecac., in 2 ounces of water, a teaspoonful every ½ hour, until nausea was produced. In the evening she was considerably relieved, having taken 6 doses of Ipecac., and being completely nauseated, the pain occurred at more distant intervals, and the flooding had nearly ceased; in a few days, the menorrhagia passed entirely off, and she recovered her usual health. For several successive periods she pursued this plan, and at the end of 6 months Menstruration was performed so naturally that she was able to lay aside entirely the use of all medicine. Dr. OSBORN also found great benefit from the use of Ipecac. WOOD says that small doses of Ipecac., repeated so as to induce slight nausea, without vomiting, will often have a happy effect in relieving vascular excitement, and controlling hæmorrhage; but vomiting will be attended with some risk of increased flowing, from the straining and consequent compression of the pelvic viscera which attend the act of vomiting. VOGT says that it has been much used in hæmorrhages, especially in metrorrhagia and spitting of blood. It has been supposed to possess a peculiar styptic power, and to exert a specific action upon the female sexual organs, because it exerts a beneficial action upon many spasmodic affections of women, arising from disorder of the menstrual and sexual functions. VOGT thinks it most useful when the bleeding arises from irritation of the nerves, rather than from an *Erethismus vasorum*, and is occasioned by abdominal disease, connected with relaxation of the tissues.

It will be seen that Ipecac. is deemed by some old school physicians to be most useful in spasmodic hæmorrhagia, and other spasmodic affections; yet its principal action is to cause a spasmodic action of the stomach and diaphragm in vomiting; while PEREIRA (see Materia Med.) gives several instances in which it caused spasmodic asthma. VOGT recommends it in spasmodic bleedings from the lungs, although he admits that it may cause irritation of the air tubes, hoarseness, cough, spitting of blood, and oppression of the chest, with inflammatory congestion of the air tubes, and congestion of the lungs. As early as 1846, I published, in the Homœopathic Examiner, new series, vol. 1, p. 407, an essay upon the spasmodic affections, especially of the lungs, caused by Ipecac.

Dose.—The 1st dilution has been successful in some cases. NOACK advises 1 or 2 drops of the pure tincture, or of the 1st and 2d dilution, every ½, 1, or 2 hours in severe cases; every 3, 4, or 6 hours in less severe attacks; or from 2 to 5 granules may be given as often. In BEAUVAIS' cases, Ipec. was used only twice, viz., in one case in the

2d dilution, in the other in the 3d ; the second dilution checked in the course of an hour a profuse flooding after miscarriage. BIGEL was in the habit of relying upon it, with much confidence.

KREOSOTE.

LEADAM recommends this remedy where there is a discharge of a large quantity of dark blood, followed for some days by the exudation of a bloody ichor, with a pungent odor, attended with corrosive itching and smarting of the parts, succeeded again by flooding, with expulsion of coagulated pieces of blood, accompanied with buzzing in the ears, and pressing pain in the head.

Kreosote has generally been regarded as a styptic remedy, from its power of coagulating the albumen of eggs and of the blood ; concentrated albuminous liquids are immediately coagulated by it ; diluted ones gradually, but fibrin is not altered by it. PEREIRA makes no mention of any specific action upon the uterine organs, but says that its influence upon the urinary organs is sometimes very marked; McLEOD and ELLIOTSON have seen the urine acquire a blackish color from its use; occasionally, it increases the quantity of urine, but in diabetes it sometimes has an opposite effect; in some instances, it causes micturition and strangury, so that its action in this respect bears some resemblance to that of Turpentine. PEREIRA says, that it acts as a most efficient styptic, partly in consequence of its power of coagulating albuminous liquids, and thereby causing the formation of a clot, and partly by causing contraction of the bleeding vessels. WOOD and BACHE say, that it will stop capillary hæmorrhage, but possesses no power to arrest bleeding from large vessels ; probably because it merely coagulates the albumen of the blood, without acting upon the fibrin. From the good effects which it has often exerted upon indolent, gangrenous, syphilitic, scrofulous and cancerous ulcers, it may also prove useful in ulcerations of the neck of the womb. VOGT says that Kreosote often increases the secretion of urine, perspiration, and the menses. Still he says that the *Aqua Binelli*, which contains impure Kreosote, has often been used with good effect against bleeding from the nose, blood-spitting, bleeding from the bowels, kidneys, and uterus.

Dose.—Noack recommends 1 or 2 drop doses, of the 1st, 2d, or 3d dilution, repeated every 2, 4, 6, 8, 12, or 24 hours. It may also be used as a vaginal injection, when the discharge is offensive, and there is ulceration of the neck of the womb.

LYCOPODIUM

Is recommended by Loomis, when there is an irritable condition of the womb, attended with chronic dryness of the vagina, and when the menses appear too early, are too profuse, and continue too long, being preceded by shivering, sadness, melancholy, and disposition to weep, or by headache, pain in the loins, fainting, and vomiting of sour substances, especially if a yellowish, milky, or reddish corrosive leucorrhœa be present during the interval.

According to Vogt, Lycopodium has frequently been used as a palliative remedy in spasmodic and inflammatory affections of the urinary and genital organs, but in large doses, viz., as much as 20 or 30 grains; from the mildness of its action, it is, however, more frequently used as a dusting powder in excoriations of children, or for enveloping pills to prevent their adhesion. Dierbach says, it has been recommended as a quieting and soothing remedy in diseases of children; especially in colic, also in whooping cough, oppression of the chest, asthmatic attacks, hysterics, cramp of the stomach, in dysuria, strangury, and gravel; as an aqua distillati Lycopodii was formerly used against stone and gravel; but it was prepared from the whole plant, and not merely from the powder. It was once a favorite domestic remedy against pains in the stomach and bowels in children. Of course it may also be used in females, when some or any of the above affections occur in connection with frequent and profuse Menstruation. Sobernheim says that in latter times, (i. e., since Hahnemann's time,) Lycopodium has been again brought forward as an excellent remedy against dysuria, retention of urine, and spasms of the bladder, especially in teething children; the whole plant has been used successfully against all degrees of ischuria, even when attended with a suppurative, or calculous condition of the urinary organs. JAHR, from abundant experience, has found it a sedative and antispasmodic remedy, well calculated to allay morbid nervous sensibility and irritation.

Dose.—NOACK advises 1 or 2 drops, per dose, of the 1st, 2, or 3d dilution, every 2, 4, 6, 8, 12, or 24 hours, according to the severity of the symptoms.

MERCURIUS

Is recommended by LOOMIS, if there be dry heat with congestion to the head, just before Menstruation; or, if during it, the tongue be red, with deep colored spots upon it, attended with a burning and salt taste in the mouth; if there be a purulent and corrosive leucorrhœa, with itching in the parts, or if there is a sensation of excoriation, with swelling of the vagina, frequent desire to urinate, painful discharge of scanty urine, of a dark color and offensive smell.

WHITEHEAD thinks, that Mercury may be homœopathic to precocious Menstruation in scrofulous females; at least he gives a case in which a girl began to menstruate at 11 years of age, after taking 20 or 30 pills containing calomel; the result was intense salivation, and she was confined to bed for 6 weeks, during which time Menstruation commenced; her health was only imperfectly restored at the end of 16 months, but from the time of its first accession, Menstruation continued to recur at regular intervals, the discharge, however, being small in quantity, pale, and attended with more or less inconvenience. Between her 13th and 17th years, she was several times affected with chlorosis, and suffered repeatedly from abscesses in the neck and arm pit, rheumatism of the head and limbs, nodes upon the legs, and mercurial salt-rheum. She was in perfect health before she took the Mercury, and neither she or any of her family had previously had any signs of scrofula; the Mercury was obviously the cause also of the early appearance of the menses, the other female members of her family having had the change at a much later period of life. She married, and transmitted the scrofulo-mercurial taint to her children in a decided form.

Dose.—1 or 2 grains per dose, of the 2d, 3d, or 6th dilution. Merc. corros. should be preferred when there is ulceration of the womb, and may also be used as a vaginal injection, 2 or 3 times a day. Very susceptible persons may use the globules.

PLATINA.

Loomis and Leadam recommend this remedy when the menses are too early, too profuse, and too long continued, attended with pressure and bearing down towards the genital organs, which are very sensitive; and if, in addition to an irritable uterus, there be induration of the womb, or congestion, especially if the discharge be of thick, dark colored, but uncoagulated blood; when there is a pressing pain, extending from the small of the back to the groins, a forcing downwards and outwards, with great excitability and tenderness of the uterus and vagina.

According to Rückert, Platina has been found useful in cases of violent hæmorrhage after miscarriage, the blood coming off in large clots; also when the flowing is attended with unnatural tenderness and sensitiveness of the genital organs, with excessive sexual desire. Also in profuse Menstruation, with discharge of thick, dark, coagulated blood, with pain in the small of the back, moving down into both groins, and causing a severe pressing down pain, with excessive tenderness and sensitiveness of the parts involved. It also cured a case in which there were severe cutting pains in the abdomen, for several days previous to Menstruation, with heavy pressing down upon the genital organs, and labor-like pains, extending from the small of the back, through the groins, into the thighs.

Dose.—The 6th and 12th dilutions have been used successfully. Madden found the 3d, 6th, and 12th potencies useful; and applied the 1st and 3d dilution of Platinum Chlor. locally to the uterus and vagina, in the form of injections; by these means he cured 11 cases out of 15, of menorrhogia. Of Beauvais' 106 cases, it was used in 4; in 1 case, in the 2d dilution, with some success; in another case, also in the 2d dilution, it cured, in 3 days, a flow which had lasted 4 or 5 weeks; —there was some aggravation on the 1st day af treatment; a 3d case, which had continued 3 weeks under allopathic treatment, was cured by 2 doses of Platina; KNORRE found it generally useful in profuse Menstruation.

PULSATILLA.

LEADAM says, although this is so important a remedy in amenorrhœa, it is nevertheless very useful at times in menorrhagia, when the blood is thick and black, or pale and watery, and flows by fits and starts; or when it is profuse, especially at the critical age, and attended with headache, noise in the ears, sadness and melancholy, and great irritation of the nerves. LOOMIS uses almost the same words, but adds, that it is also indicated when there is an irritable uterus, with pains in the loins, shiverings, dizziness, tenesmus of the rectum and bladder, scanty red or brown urine, with frequent desire to urinate, before, during, or after the monthly period, and a thick, corrosive, burning leucorrhœa. In my opinion, Pulsatilla is more homœopathic to menorrhagia than to amenorrhœa (see North American Journal of Homœopathy, vol. 1, p. 196); VOGT and DIERBACH think that it acts so powerfully upon the kidney, uterus, and rectum, that suppressed hæmorrhoids and menses reappear during its use. According to RÜCKERT, it is useful in metrorrhagia when the flow is not continuous, but ceases at times, in order to return again with increased violence, much coagulated blood being evacuated. Also when menorrhagia with false labor-pains, occur in pregnant females, the blood being blackish and clotted at times, at others liquid, the vagina being contracted and dry, so that it could only be examined with pain and difficulty; when the patient is exhausted by pain and flowing, and the pains do not force the uterus to contract. It also relieved a violent flooding after confinement, from adhesion of the placenta.

Dose.—MADDEN used the 1st, 3d, 6th, and 12th dilutions of Pulsatilla; the 200th dilution was thought to be useful in 2 cases. NOACK advises 1 or 2 drops, per dose, of the pure tincture, or of the 1st, 2d, 3d, or 6th dilution, to be repeated frequently in some cases, but only once or twice a day in less urgent attacks; still he prefers the second dilution as a rule, as he thinks that it has proved more successful in his hands than any other preparation of this remedy. Delicate and sensitive persons may take 2 or 3 globules per dose, as often as above recommended. In BEAUVAIS' 106 cases, Pulsat. was used in 5; in one case each, the 18th and 30th dilutions produced little or no good effect; the 12th seemed to check the flow, in one case, in 12 minutes; the 15th relieved one case in ½ hour, which had continued for 15 days; the 4th dilution was used in another case.

SABINA,

According to LOOMIS, is one of the most prominent homœopathic remedies for profuse Menstruation, when it results from an irritable uterus, especially about the period of the change of life, and is connected with irregularity as to time; the discharge being profuse, consisting of clotted or bright red blood, attended with pains, like those of labor, in the loins and groins, and contracting pains about the womb, and by an itching, yellowish, fetid leucorrhœa. It is all the more indicated if the mouth of the womb be more open than usual, the lips swollen, and neck tender. LEADAM thinks it is most indicated when there is a discharge of black, dark colored, and clotted blood, with labor-pains in the loins and womb; or where there are paroxysmal discharges of bright red blood, increased by motion, especially in women who have frequently suffered from abortion, and who have reached that age when the change of life should occur. According to RÜCKERT, Sabina cured a case of metrorrhagia which had lasted for 11 weeks, there being a great discharge of black blood, and frequently of large coagulæ, especially at night, although the show was often of a bright red; there were violent tearing pains in the limbs, in the small of the back, and in the abdomen; also a tearing headache, generally on the left side, and frequently of intolerable severity. Also a severe case with labor-like pains, moving from the small of the back to the groins, and excessive urging to urinate. A third case, recurring after a miscarriage, the blood being generally coagulated, dark, and blackish, or, more rarely, thin and watery; at night the flow lessened and was painless; at other times there was a pressure above the pubis, and a bearing down upon the womb; also general weakness, emaciation, pallor and vertigo. Also a chronic case with severe and peculiar pains in the limbs. And a fifth case, attended with griping pains in the abdomen, the blood being thin, and the patient very weak. The 1st, 5th, 8th, and 30th dilutions were all used with good effect.

According to PEREIRA's experience, it is the most certain and powerful emmenagogue in the whole Materia Medica; its emmenagogue power is fully established, the observations of HOME being perhaps the most satisfactory of any on this subject, confirmed, as they are, by the reports of many other accurate observers. It has acted so violently upon the kidneys and bladder, that bloody urine has been passed, and coagulated blood found in the bladder. In excessive cases, it has caused violent and incessant vomiting, excruciating pains in the womb, followed by abortion, and dreadful hæmorrhage; after death, the gall-bladder has been found ruptured, the bile effused into the abdomen, and the intestines inflamed, and all this perhaps from a specific action upon the liver, as it causes an increased secretion of bile, and increase of size of the liver; hence it is homœopathic to menorrhagia, when connected with bilious derangement, and portal congestion. WOOD and BACHE say that it increases most of the secretions, especially those of the skin and womb, to the latter of which organs it is supposed to have a peculiar direction, so that it has been much used in amenorrhœa. In pregnancy it should be given with much caution, although it has recently been recommended as an effective remedy in certain forms of menorrhagia, and is asserted to prove occasionally useful in preventing threatened abortion (see Am. Jour. Med. Sciences, new series, vol. 8, p. 475). DIERBACH says that it readily causes congestion of blood to the genital organs, increases the urine, and in large doses even causes hæmaturia. He recommends it in chronic and feverless affections of the womb, in suppression of the menses, sterility, swelling of the womb, in consequence of frequent pregnancies, in cramps of the womb, subsequent to frequent miscarriages, in leucorrhœa, chronic hæmorrhages from the uterus, and even in indurations and commencing cancerous degeneration of this organ; also in blenorrhœas of the genital organs of both sexes. Vogt says that it removes sluggishness, stagnation, and thickness of the vena porta blood, and increases, in an especial degree, the sanguineous congestion and secretion from the uterus, while, at the same time, it is the most efficient of all the balsams, in removing sluggishness, relaxation, and atony of the womb. That it excels, in its action upon the female genital organs, all other gum-resins and balsams is undoubted by all sound practitioners, and it is the more indicated in diseases of these organs, the more languor there is of their vessels and movements, the more torpor in the ganglionic system, and the more atony and relaxation there is in general. He also recommends it highly against profuse, too frequently returning, and too long continuing Menstruation, arising from simple atony of the uterus.

In the American Jour. of Med. Sciences, Oct., 1844, p. 475, we learn that some observations on the employment of the Juniperus Sabina, in hæmorrhage from the uterus, have been made by M. Aran, from which it would seem to be occasionally a powerful agent in *checking* these discharges. Much has been said on the properties of Savin as an emmenagogue; several foreign authors, however, and among them, Wedekind, Günther, and Santer, disregard altogether its tendency to *cause* uterine hæmorrhage, and, on the contrary, recommend its use in such cases. M. Santer says that Sabina is one of the most powerful curative means, not only in menorrhagia, but also in those hæmorrhages which threaten abortion, occurring in pregnant women, who, from debility, have already had several miscarriages. He states that in these cases he had given the powder of Sabina, in the extraordinary doses of 15 to 20 grains, three times a day, during a period of 3, 4, or even 5 months, and that he has in this manner frequently succeeded in arresting the flowing, and preventing abortion, the infants being born healthy, at the full period.

The following cases, among others, are mentioned by ARAN:

CASE 1.—A worker in embroidery, aged 33, had been recently delivered of a child, and since her confinement had had attacks of menorrhagia at irregular intervals; she was much debilitated, and her health began to fail. Powdered Savin was given; in two days the flowing ceased, and did not return again.

CASE 2.—A woman, aged 28, had suffered from menorrhagia, almost continually for eight months; Sabina was given, and on the 3d day the bleeding was arrested. About six weeks afterwards, the flow returned, Sabina was again given, and the bleeding ceased almost immediately.

CASE 3.—A robust lady was attacked with menorrhagia, after a fatiguing walk; it was neglected, and had already lasted several days; 1¼ gramme (about 20 grains) of Savin was administered in 3 doses, and on the following day the bleeding had ceased, and, although the patient would not remain in bed, it did not again return.

CASE 4.—A young married lady was attacked at the menstrual period with profuse flowing, which had continued for 8 days; 3 doses of Savin, of 40 centigrammes each, were given at intervals of 2 hours; on the following day the hæmorrhage had almost ceased, and another dose of the medicine entirely put a stop to it.

The celebrated KOPP has found Sabina useful in active uterine hæmorrhage, and prides himself not a little upon his discovery. SANTER expressly confines his use of it to passive hæmorrhages, and all diseases of the uterus depending on atony, asthenia, debility, defect of contractility, or cohesive force in uterus.

In Franks' Magazine, we also find Sabina recommended against profuse Menstruation and menorrhagia, by old school physicians, in allopathic doses.

CASE 5.—A very poor woman, aged 40, who had had several children and abortions, suffered with profuse Menstruation, lasting from 6 to 8 days; the blood was almost as black as coffee, and exceedingly offensive; every time before the menses set in, her breath became very offensive, and the womb was found enlarged to the size of a child's head, and projected above the pubis; it diminished in size during the flow; the patient had many hysterical symptoms, and was pale, and discolored. After an abortion a flowing commenced, and lasted for 6 weeks, her pulse became small and quick, and fever set in. Twenty-grain doses of Sabina were given, 4 times a day, and quickly restored her; afterwards she always took a *small* (?) dose of Sabina, every night and morning, for 4 days, before the recurrence of Menstruation, with such good effect, that the menses always sat in without pain or distress, and were no longer profuse. She recovered her health and strength entirely.—WEDEKIND.

CASES 6 and 7.—In 2 cases of bleeding from the womb, in women who were approaching the change of life, and which had withstood all the ordinary treatment, Sabina was given successfully in scruple doses, and more, 4 times a day. Hence, although this remedy is an emmenagogue, it must also be regarded as among the best styptics against bleeding from the womb, but only in cases of true atomy and torpidity of the womb.—GÜNTHER.

CASE 8.—A delicate and nervous woman, aged 36, who had had many children, had also suffered for years with pain in the kidneys and bladder; after a suppression of 3 months, Menstruation sat in profusely; blood was discharged in thick, coagulated pieces, with violent labor-like pains in the back, but no signs of a fœtus were found. The discharge, which was at first bright red, then dark and coagulated, had already lasted profusely for 10 days, and the patient began to have frequent fainting fits; finally, the flow became brownish and granular, like decayed cruor, gave forth a horrible stench, like that of putrid meat, and that so powerfully, that it was difficult to remain in the room.

Treatment.—After many other remedies had failed, 3 drachms of Fol. Sabin. were infused in 4 ounces of water, and a tablespoonful given every two hours. The discharge altered after the 2d dose, and was somewhat increased in quantity, but in an hour more it began to lessen, the offensive smell improved, and the pain in the groins ceased. In the course of 4 days, all offensive odor had disappeared, and the discharge ceased gradually.

CASE 9.—A lady began to have such profuse Menstruation that she was obliged to remain in bed for several days each month, and always lost a large quantity of blood. Appropriate homœopathic remedies, among which were Sabina, 3d and 6th dilutions, were given without good effect; then 3 drachms of Fol. Sabin. were infused in 6 ounces of water, and a tablespoonful given every 2 hours, with rapid and permanent benefit. —KOPP.

Dose.—The 1st, 5th, 8th, and 30th dilutions have each proved successful, or, at least, cases of menorrhagia have subsided under their use. MADDEN used the 3d and 6th dilutions, of the decimal scale. The doses must be repeated every ½, 1, or 2 hours, in very urgent cases; 2 or 3 times a day in, less severe attacks. Very impressible patients may take from 2, or 3, to 5 granules per dose. In BEAUVAIS' 106 cases, Sabina was used more frequently and successfully than any other remedy, viz., in 16 cases; viz., the 2d dilut. in 1 case; the 3d relieved 1 case in a month, which had already lasted a month; also, another case in 1½ hours, which had continued several hours; the 6th and 7th dilutions each in 1 case; the 8th dilution checked a flow in 2 days, which had persisted for 14 days; the 12th potency was used in 1 case; the 24th in another; the 30th relieved 1 case in 2 days, which had continued for 11 weeks; finally, a part of a grain of the powder relieved a a case in 3 days, which had lasted only 1 day.

SECALE.

LEADAM says that Secale is, as might be supposed, a valuable agent in menorrhagia; it is indicated in the congestive form, when the menses are profuse, especially at the climacteric period; in weak, cachectic, and exhausted individuals, with cold extremities, pale face, small pulse, and with anxiety and despondency. He says it should be used in the low attenuations. CHURCHILL says, that Secale will increase if not originate uterine contractions, is known to all, and also that it will restrain inordinate discharges from the womb; we should, however, scarcely expect it to be useful in exciting the menstrual secretion, and it is difficult to determine upon what principle it does so. (Homœopathy will explain it.) As to the fact, we have the evidence of DEWEES, who recommends its use; of Dr. LOCOCK, who has tried it with success; also ROCHE, NAUCHE, and PAULY.

Dose.—In uterine hæmorrhage this remedy should almost always be used in massive doses; still, MADDEN gave the 3d, 6th, and 30th dilutions of the decimal scale. It may be given every few minutes in very urgent cases; every few hours in less severe attacks; and once or twice a day in chronic states. In BEAUVAIS' cases, it was used in 4.

SULPHUR

Is recommended by LOOMIS, when there is a painful sensibility of the neck and body of the womb, attended by itching and a burning sensation in the parts, before the menses set in. Or, when there is headache, spasmodic colic, pressure on the part, restlessness, cough, heart-burn, bleeding from the nose, and yellowish corrosive leucorrhœa, especially if Menstruation recurs too early, and is too profuse, or the blood is too pale, and has an acid smell. In all chronic cases of long standing, it will be well to commence the treatment with Sulphur; LOOMIS has known a dose or two of Sulphur change the whole character of the case; in nearly all cases which he has treated successfully with Sulphur, there has been a quick pulse, flushed cheek, hot skin, frequent attacks of headache, high-colored, scanty, and fetid urine, with a greasy pellicle on its surface, and passed with pain. It is more frequently indicated during the interval, than at the menstrual period.

Dose.—MADDEN used the 3d, 6th, and 12th dilutions.

VERATRUM

Is recommended by LEADAM, when frequent and profuse Menstruation is attended with diarrhœa, especially when there is buzzing in the ears, bleeding from the nose, pain in all the limbs, and great thirst.

THLAPSI BURSA PASTORIS

Is recommenned by Dr. LANGE, who has noticed the greatest benefit from this plant, in the menorrhagies of persons of relaxed constitutions; he has often cured entirely the tendency to excessive discharges at the menstrual periods.

EMMENAGOGUES.

These remedies, of course, are homœopathic to menorrhagia, in addition to those already mentioned. DIERBACH mentions the Taxus baccata, Laurus nobilis, Ruta graveolens, Buchu, Asarum europæum, and Borax.

He says, that *Taxus baccata* has frequently caused fetid smelling sweats, with itching of the skin and pustular eruptions, flow of mucus and blood from the sexual organs, increased secretion of urine, diarrhœa, flow of viscid and acrid spittle, and attacks of vertigo, with dimness of vision. Hence it may prove homœopathic in scrofulous cases, with obstinate eruptions of the skin and acne, bad-smelling perspirations from the skin, arm-pits, perinæum, and feet, with leucorrhœa and tendency to diarrhœa.

The *Laurus nobilis* is most indicated when there is a tendency to abortion.

The *Rue* is most indicated when there are fetid sweats and hæmaturia.

Buchu is most homœopathic when there is a tendency to profuse secretion of urine, the water being turbid, loaded with flocculi, and presenting a purulent appearance; also, in dysmenorrhœa, leucorrhœa, and chronic menorrhagia, when attended with symptoms of gravel, great irritability of the bladder, with thickening, ulceration, or catarrh of the bladder.

Asarum europæum is one of the most common and active remedies in the production of abortion.

The emmenagogue action of Borax is said to be undoubted.

Senega is most useful when there is a decided catarrhal affection of the chest.

Nitre, by stimulating the kidneys, is said to be a decided emmenagogue. ASHWELL gave it to a patient whose mother placed great confidence in it, in scruple doses, 3 or 4 times daily, in a wineglass of water; it purged and produced bloody motions, but on the 3d day there was a copious flow of the menses, after a suppression of 7 months.

In BEUVAIS' 106 cases, besides the remedies already mentioned, Nux was given in 7 cases, Arsen., Baryt. c., Carb. an., Sepia, Silex, and Sulph., each in 1 case.

DELAYED MENSTRUATION.

OF 4,000 cases, WHITEHEAD, of Manchester, met with

499	which	were	delayed	to the	17th	year.
393	"	"	"	"	18	"
148	"	"	"	"	19	"
71	"	"	"	"	20	"
20	"	"	"		21st or 26	"

WHITEHEAD found that delayed Menstruation and puberty exerted a more unfavorable influence than precocity; precocious cases were attended with unfavorable symptoms in about 20 per cent.; when puberty was delayed to the 17th or 18th year, as many as 247 cases out of 892, or about 28 per cent., presented unfavorable symptoms; while nearly 41 per cent., or 97 cases out of 239, who menstruated for the first time at 19 years of age, or after, required careful medical attendance, not so much for the absent discharge, as for their general health.

From the table (see page 9,) it will be seen that in *cold* climates it is almost as natural for women to commence to menstruate as late as 22 years, as at 14 years of age; while very few, only 19 out of 6745 cases commence as early as 13 years; only 5 cases out of 6745, at 12 years; and only 1 case out of 6745, at 11 years of age. Hence, protection from cold is very important for girls suffering with delayed or scanty Menstruation; exposure to warmth, either by means of exceedingly warm clothing, warm houses, or a residence in a warm climate, necessarily becomes an exceedingly effectual agent in the treatment of these cases, although exceedingly precocious Menstruation is not as common in hot climates as is generally supposed. In Venezuela the menses set in, only in very rare cases, as early as 10 years of age.

Only 10 per cent. commence at 11 or 12 years.

As many as 70 per cent. commence from 13 to 15 years.

About 20 per cent. commence as late as 16 to 18 years.

And very rare cases, from 19 to 20 years, or even 21 years.

Still, in the large majority of women in *hot* climates, the changes of puberty are accomplished before the 15th year; in *temperate* climates, from the 13th to the 18th year; and in *cold* climates, from the 14th to the 22d year.

If Menstruation be delayed beyond the usual period, TILT says, nothing can be plainer than the line of conduct a mother should adopt in reference to her daughter's health;—if she be well, however late the first appearance may be delayed, no *physic* is required;—if she be ill, medical advice should be sought. The mother should recollect that puberty occurs at different periods, according to the country, climate, class of society, and even the constitution, and in many cases, it is safely delayed many years beyond the usual time. The knowledge that this may happen, without serious detriment to the health of the girl, should be sufficient to prevent the infatuation of so many well-intentioned mothers, who, merely because the "custom of women" has not appeared in their daughters at the same age as it appeared in themselves, do not hesitate to administer forcing medicines, without asking the sanction of a medical opinion.

The following sad history, related by Dr. DEWEES, is, TILT says, the best case that can be given on this subject.

"I often call to mind, with bitter recollection, the fate of a most amiable and interesting creature, for whom I was requested to prescribe for the expected menses, but who had not one mark that could justify an interference, more especially as she was in perfectly good health. 'She was fifteen; it was time'; and this was all that could be urged by the mother in favor of an attempt 'to bring down the courses.' I relied too much on the good sense of her anxious parent, and fully explained myself to her, without prescribing for her child. As might be expected, she determined upon trying a quack medicine, of some celebrity in similar cases; in a few days her daughter became feverish, lost her appetite, and suffered from nausea; she was soon confined to her bed, and by a persistence in the same treatment, she soon lost an only and a lovely daughter."

The line of conduct to be pursued by the physician when consulted about a case of retarded or delayed Menstruation, is equally plain. It should be recollected, and explained, that many girls do not come to maturity of mind and body as early as others; if the health of the child be generally good, her mind and body, however, being rather immature, then the principal attention should be paid to the development and culture of the *physique* and *morale*, rather than to a merely one-sided regard for the menstrual function. Menstruation should only be encouraged when both mind and body are prepared for it, and for the duties, precautions, and feelings, which attend it; a mere child is not fit to be entrusted with all the attributes, or to have the functions of mature women thrust upon her.

Excessively studious and sedentary habits should be corrected; exercise on foot and in a carriage, riding on horseback, sea bathing, the games of battledore, jumping the rope, rolling the hoop, running, and particularly dancing, are powerful means for obtaining health of body and vigor of mind, which ought not to be neglected, and which fortunately women seldom object to putting in practice. Living in the country, for the summer season at least, where the air is pure, particularly if pleasant company and companions can be added to the charms afforded by diversity of views and landscapes. Pic-nics, riding and boating excursions, evening entertainments, &c., which unite to all the advantages of exercises that of being agreeable to young persons, and producing the useful stimulus of contact with older and maturer minds of both sexes, will rapidly and healthily mature a feeble body, and one-sided, or torpid mind. All these means should be aided by a carefully selected, nourishing, and rather hearty diet; young girls should be methodically and carefully discouraged from acquiring morbid inclinations for sickening and debilitating trash, miscalled delicacies; for they too soon get a distaste for all really nourishing and strengthening food.

The medical treatment should be calculated to produce the same broad and comprehensive changes, which nature designed to do, and which the above hygienic treatment may fail to accomplish. The physician should recollect that a proportionately more rapid growth and development of the whole body, more extended powers of mind and imagination, vigor of form and carriage, and the bloom of health and beauty, should be accomplished either by nature, or by the medical and hygienic arts; and that a contemptible and irritating treatment of a few organs or parts, is but little calculated to accomplish these great changes.

INFREQUENT MENSTRUATION.

Madden, in 181 cases of uterine derangement, met with 9 cases in which Menstruation was infrequent; Whitehead, in 161 cases of irregular Menstruation, found 5 cases in which the returns generally happened every 5 or 6 weeks, but occasionally there was an interval of only 1 month; one lady generally had her courses monthly, but every 3d time she missed the period, having a free interval of 2 months, her health never suffering in consequence. Colombat says, some women naturally only have their "turns" every 6 weeks, or even only every 2 months; Linnæus saw women in Lapland, whose periodical discharges occurred only once a year; Lisfranc has met with women who were regular every 5th or 6th month, or only every 4th or 6th year; some of these females were habitually disordered, and others enjoyed perfect health. Colombat thinks that girls of a lymphatic or scrofulous constitution, are regulated later and with more difficulty than others; while scrofulous women who are already regulated, often find their menstrual discharges diminishing little by little, and the retardations constantly becoming more prolonged.

Although we have seen that many mothers are too anxious for the first appearance of Menstruation in their daughters, still, an equally large class are too inattentive to the proper regulation and periodical occurrence of this function; nothing is more common than to meet with girls who have their periods at long intervals only, and then unsatisfactorily, but who do not get medical attendance until some severe accidental disease renders it imperatively necessary that their health should be attended to. Then the physician is obliged to contend with the complicated effects of a badly regulated system, conjoined with acute disease, and the constant liability to relapses, and various unusual occurrences, which are apt to arise in this state of things.

Treatment of Delayed and Infrequent Menstruation.

SULPHUR

Is supposed to act specifically upon the venous system of the abdomen, lower bowels, and pelvis; ALTSCHUL says, it causes congestion to the womb, with pressing-down pains, and tendency to inflammation of the vulva, the menses occurring either too early or too profusely, or else being suppressed in consequence of inflammation, or irritation. KNORRE, however, recommends it when there suppression of the menses, with congestion of blood to the head; in falling of the womb, leucorrhœa, and inclination to abortion. It has also been decided to be homœopathic when Menstruation occurs at too late a period, and too infrequently, attended with constipation and distension of the abdomen, even when there is a delay of 3 months beyond the usual time.

Dose.—NOACK advises 1 or 2 grains of the 1st or 3d trituration, or from 1 to 3 drops of a carefuly prepared tinct. of Sulphur, repeated once or twice a day, or every 2, 4, or 6 days.

NATRUM.

Natrum sulph. has been recommended when the menses are delayed beyond the usual time, being too late in their first occurrence, infrequent in their recurrence, and scanty, with constipation. *Natrum muriaticum*, when they are simply too late and scanty. Natrum is supposed to exert a specific action upon the neck, the genital organs especially in the female sex, upon the tissues of the womb, upon the urinary organs, and breast; it has also removed goitre, and other affections of the cervical glands. *Natrum carb. acidulum* has removed enlarged cervical glands, scrofulous derangement of the stomach and bowels. The Chlorate of Soda has removed irregularity of Menstruation in scrofulous females, with enlargements of the glands of the neck. The Iodide of Soda has removed tumors which have withstood the use of Iod. mer., and Iod. pot.

Dose.—1 or 2 grains of the 1st, 2d, 3d, or 6th *decimal* dilution, may be taken night and morning, or every 2, 3, or 4 days; in appropriate cases, and in very sensitive persons, from 2 to 5 granules may be taken per dose.

CHELIDONIUM

Has been recommended when the menses are retarded and infrequent as to time, but last longer, and are more profuse in quantity. It has effected cures in women afflicted with obstinate eruptions upon the face, with most extensive and profuse scrofulous ulcerations, and with bilious derangement.

Dose.—NOACK advises 1 or 2 drop doses of the pure tincture, repeated once or twice a day. The granules may be used in very nervous, hysterical, and sensitive persons.

SABADILLA

Has been used successfully when Menstruation is delayed and infrequent, and is preceded for several days by a painful bearing-down; it is most useful in cases in which there is a frequent inclination to urinate, drawing pains along the spine, chilliness of the body, with a peculiar feeling of warmth in abdomen, and a characteristic sensation of excessive debility.

Dose.—1 or 2 drops of the 1st, 2d, or 3d dilution, may be used per dose; or from 2 to 4 granules.

NUX MOSCHATA

Is recommended in infrequent and tardy Menstruation, when preceded by a severe and peculiar pain in the back, especially if many hysterical and nervous symptoms be present, such as delirium, vertigo, hysterical loss of sensation, drowsiness, or transient mental derangement.

Dose.—Same as for Chelidonium.

MERCURIALIS PERENNIS

Has been used when there was a delay of 3 days, and the menses then set in with a sense of anxiety, difficult breathing, feverish heat over the whole body, followed by swelling and tenderness of the breasts, headache, and faintness, especially if these symptoms occur in girls who are usually light and happy, sprightly, gay, and merry, but who become feverish, surly, fretful, sullen, and depressed, or excited, with dizziness and drowsiness, heaviness, fulness, heat, and congestion of the head. It is homœopathic when the menses, which should last at least 3 days, continue only 1 day, followed by cramps in the bowels, and headache; also, when the menses are delayed for 1 week; when they last only 4 days, scantily, in females in whom they generally continue 7 days.

Dose.—Same as given for Sabadilla. (page 78.)

MAGNESIA MURIATICA,

When there is a delay in Menstruation, with violent pain in the small of the back.

Dose.—The same as recommended for Natrum. (page 78.)

IODINE

Is recommended as homœopathic, when there is a delay in Menstruation, with dizziness and palpitation; still, ASHWELL says, that it is occasionally a good emmenagogue, but also, that there is no remedy of this class, which has so frequently failed in his hands;* in patients predisposed to struma, or actually suffering from scrofulous enlargements of the glands, it exerts an almost specific influence; still Coindet was perhaps scarcely correct in attributing to this drug such certain and powerful emmenagogue properties. Churchill says, that Iodine has been extensively tried in amenorrhœa, and in many cases successfully; but it may be questioned whether the continued trial has fulfilled the expectation of the physician who introduced it into practice. Colombat says, that Iodine has been used successfully in chronic amenorrhœa, by Coindet, Dumeril, Brera of Padua, Magendie, Sablairolet, Recamier, and Trousseau, as well as by himself. But Dr. Manson does not believe that it possesses any emmenagogue powers, further than as a stimulant and tonic to the whole body; in one of his patients, in large doses, it occasioned so much sickness and disorder of the stomach, that the menstrual discharge was suppressed altogether. It has been supposed to be most useful in irregular Menstruation, arising from enlargement or induration of the womb; Dr. Thetford gave it in a case in which the uterus was of bony hardness, and of so considerable a size as nearly to fill the whole of the pelvis; yet in six weeks the disease had given way to the use of Iodine, and Menstruation was restored. Ashwell treated successfully 7 cases of hard tumors of the womb, in the average time of from 8 to 16 weeks. Lugol mentions several instances among his scrofulous patients, in which it cured obstructed and painful Menstruation. Eager found it to act as an excitant on the genital organs; it augmented the activity of the womb, and rendered Menstruation more abundant; on the other hand it has been supposed to be homœopathic to sterility, as 2 cases are detailed by Dr. Rob. H. Rivers, in which barrenness succeeded its administration. Locher Balber found Iodine of use, at times, in those troublesome cases, which occasionally precede the establishment of Menstruation, but if given in too large doses, he and Golis were often obliged to omit its use, on account of its evil consequences to the lungs, such as dry cough, and cough with bloody expectoration. Dierbach says, that Iodine may cause an atrophic state of the female breasts, and its influence upon the womb may stand in a more or less close connection with this power; hence he can scarcely regard it as a contradiction, when one observer notices sterility to follow its use, while another finds it to be a powerful emmenagogue, easily exciting profuse flooding, or even abortion. In a woman, subject to profuse Menstruation every 3 weeks, SCHMIDT noticed a violent flowing from the womb, lasting 4 weeks, produced by the use of Iodine. To increase the confusion caused by all these contradictory statements it has been pronounced homœopathic against sudden suppression of the flowing menses; also, when they are delayed 8 days, with vertigo and palpitation; against menstrual irregularity; increase of the menstrual flow; premature, copious, and violent Menstruation. It has *relieved* a uterine hæmorrhage, which was increased whenever the bowels were moved, attended with pains in the stomach, loins, and small of the back; it proved useful when the menses were preceded by a rush of blood to the head, palpitation of the heart, and swelling of the neck; it has also removed all the usual troublesome precursory symptoms of Menstruation. It is, perhaps, most homœopathic when scanty Menstruation is caused by congestion to the chest, in females inclined to consumption, with pains in the side, dry cough, bloody expectoration, more or less fever, and tightness of the chest, acute pains in the female breasts, as if they were sore and ulcerated in their inmost substance, continuing for weeks, and attended with painfulness and heaviness of both mammæ, followed by considerable emaciation of the whole body, or great diminution in size of the breasts.

Dose.—NOACK advises drop doses of the pure tincture, largely diluted in water, or of the 1st, 2d, 4th, or 6th dilution, once or twice a day. KNORRE advises ½ drop doses of the 1st or 3d dilution. The granules may be used in very sensitive persons.

FERRUM ACET.,

When delaying menses consist of a scanty discharge of watery blood.

DULCAMARA,

When Menstruation is retarded, with discharge of thin,

watery blood. When the menses are delayed for many days, even for 25.

Dose.—Dulcamara is one of the milder remedies, of which NOACK advises 1 or 2 drops per dose, of the pure tincture, or of the 1st or 2d dilution, from 1 to 3 times a day. In appropriate cases, the higher dilutions may be tried, or from 3 to 6 granules may be dissolved in a wineglassful of water, and 1 teaspoonful taken per dose.

SEPIA,

When the menses are three days too late.

Dose.—Same as for Natrum. (See page 78.)

CICUTA,

Late Menstruation.

Dose.—Same as for Sabadilla. (See page 78.)

HYOSC. AND IGNAT.,

When "courses" are some days too late.

Dose.—Same as for Cicuta.

PODOPHYLLUM PELT.,

When menses are retarded and infrequent.

Dose.—Same as for Dulcamara.

NUX VOM.,

When menses do not appear for 6 weeks, and then come on again at the time of full moon.

Dose.—Same as for Sabadilla.

BELLADONNA,

Increase and delay of Menstruation for 22, 36, or even 48 days.

Dose.—See page 40.

CALCAREA

Cured a case in which Menstruation was often delayed to the 6th week, but was then very profuse, attended with severe colic, frequent headache, dizziness; violent chronic cough, with pressure upon the chest, as if it were too contracted, causing her to wake several times at night, with asthma and fearfulness; she had no appetite, was very weak, gloomy, and discontented.

Dose.—Same as recommended from Natrum. (See page 78.)

GRAPHITE

Is homœopathic when the menses are delayed beyond the proper period of return. It cured a case in which Menstruation was delayed and too scanty, setting in only every 5 weeks, the patient being dizzy even when sitting, having buzzing in the ears, tearing pains in the temples, just before the monthly period, heat in the face, excessive appetite. Menstruation in this case was attended on the first day by cutting pain and pressure in the abdomen, extending down to the womb, the discharge being scanty; the patient was costive, having a hard evacuation only every 2 or 3 days; in the evening, while in bed, she often had a peculiar pain and cramp in the calves of the legs; in the morning she was so dizzy as often to be on the point of falling. It also proved useful in another case of scanty and infrequent Menstruation, in which the courses set in irregularly, only every 8 or 10 weeks, the discharge being thick and as black as pitch, being preceded and accompanied by continual headache, by cutting and pressing pains in the lower part of the stomach, and in the hips. The patient also had pain in the small of the back; the abdomen, arms, and legs were bloated, with numbness, tingling, and stinging in them, as if they would go to sleep; she was chilly, had cold hands and feet; she had rapidly grown stout, with feeling of heaviness, weariness, and inactivity; she also had small, round, red, and itching herpetic eruptions upon the forearms and neck.

Dose.—Same as for Natrum. (See page 78.)

PHOSPHORUS

Is said to be homœopathic when the menses appear too late by 4 or 8 days, but then are so much the more profuse, lasting 8 days, leaving great debility behind, the patient having dark circles around the eyes, becoming emaciated and anxious.

Dose.—Same as for Iodine. (See page 81.)

CONIUM AND KALI CARB.

Have been frequently employed with success, when the first appearance of the menses is retarded.

Dose.—Same as for Bellad. and Natrum.

SCANTY MENSTRUATION.

Whitehead, in 359 cases, met with a woman of strong and healthy constitution, whose Menstruation had commenced regularly for years, on Tuesdays, but the discharge never continued longer than 24 hours; also 8 other females, of different habits of body and differently occupied, who only menstruated one day each time. In one case, a lady had her turns every 14 days, but the discharge generally continued only 2 days, and sometimes only a few hours. Madden, in 181 cases of uterine derangement, met with 35 instances of scanty Menstruation. Although Loomis estimates the natural quantity of the menstrual flow at from 2 to 4 ounces, still, all cases in which less than from 4 to 6 ounces are parted with, must be regarded as decidedly scanty; the same holds true in all instances in which the flow lasts less than 3 or 4 days, unless it be unusually copious during that time.

Treatment of Scanty Menstruation.

BARYTA CARB.,

When the menses are simply scanty.

PULSATILLA.

In scanty Menstruation, the discharge ceasing entirely at night, and returning only in the day time while walking.

Dose.—See page 95.

SARSAPARILLA,

When the discharge is scanty and acrid, causing burning and excoriation of the inner side of the thighs.

Dose.—Same as for Pulsatilla.

IGNATIA,

When menses are scanty, black and offensive.

Dose.—Same as for Nux.

BERBERIS VULGARIS,

When the flow is scanty, also thin, like serum, setting in with chilliness, aching in the small of the back, and tearing pains in the whole body.

Dose.—Same as for Pulsatilla.

SABADILLA,

When the usually regular menses become scanty, and occur at irregular periods.

Dose.—Same as for Pulsatilla.

THUYA,

When the monthly flow is diminished and delayed.

Dose.—Same as for Pulsatilla.

DULCAMARA,

Against scanty Menstruation.

Dose.—Same as for Pulsatilla.

Bovista, Croton, Graphite, Kali carb., Lachesis, Magnesia sulph., Natrum mur., Nux, Petrol., Phos., Sepia, Baryta carb., Carb. veg., and Silex, are also recommended.

AQUILEGIA

Is said to be beneficial in many uterine affections, especially when the menses, although regular as to time, are too scanty and attended with a dull, painful, nightly increasing pressure in the right lumbar region.

Dose.—Same as for Pulsatilla.

ATRIPLEX OLIDA

Is said to have cured a case in which the menses were scanty, and generally consisted of bloody mucus, being preceded by violent lancinations and cuttings, and followed by leucorrhœa; the patient being pale and livid, having dulness of the head, constant restlessness and tossing in bed, getting but little sleep, being troubled with anxious and frightful dreams; she also had great weakness in the small of the back, especially in the afternoon, when it was at times so great as almost to cause her to sink or fall down.

Dose.—Same as for Aquilegia.

CALCAREA,

It is said, may not only be used against profuse, but also against scanty Menstruation; it is even more frequently appropriate in the latter case.

Dose.—See page 48.

GRAPHITE

Cured a case in which Menstruation had been scanty for 4 years; it was attended with colic, drawing pains in all the limbs, and by weakness. She had a cramping pain at the pit of the stomach after every meal, followed by offensive eructations; but little appetite. Baryta relieved the colic; but Graphite brought the menses on more abundantly. Graphite and Causticum are said to be useful when the appearance of the menses takes place with pain and difficulty, the discharge being scanty and soon ceasing.

Dose.—See page 96.

BARYTA CARB.,

When the menses are scanty, and last only 1 day, but set in 2 days too soon—discharge of a little bloody mucus from the vagina, with anxious beating of the heart, uneasiness in the body. According to NEUMANN, Baryta is decidedly homœopathic to torpor of the sexual system.

Dose.—Same as for Calcarea.

ALUMINA.

The action of this remedy is very similar to that of Baryta. It is homœopathic when the menses are scanty and last only 3 days; when they are scanty and pale; when suppressed for 3 months, or only for 1 month, and then set in copiously—preceded for 6 days by a copious flow of menses from the vagina, attended with trembling lassitude, and feeling as if everything would fall out—frequent urination during Menstruation, the urine being acrid—violent headache, which ceased on the appearance of the menses. Profuse and acrid leucorrhœa, with a burning sensation in the part, but especially in the rectum.

Dose.—Same as for Calcarea.

ASSAFŒTIDA.

PEREIRA.—In JÖRG's experiments it produced irritation of the sexual organs, while Menstruation appeared before its usual time, and was attended with uterine pain—it has been employed in uterine obstructions, such as amenorrhœa and chlorosis, but CULLEN very seldom succeeded with it as an emmenagogue—perhaps he might have met with better success if he had merely used it against that peculiar form of scanty and painful Menstruation which occurs too soon and frequently. SOBERNHEIM thinks, that it stands in quite a specific relation to the uterine nervous system, and there is no other remedy which so readily regulates the altered activities of the female sexual organs; it effects as much against nervous derangements of the womb, as Bismuth does in the purely nervous affections of the stomach—in menostasia and irregularity of the menses, owing to a perverse activity of the uterine nervous system, especially in delicate, badly regulated, and spasmodic girls. VOGT recommends it in atony, when attended with an irritable state of the uterine nerves; in many nervous and spasmodic affections connected with mentrual disturbances; in painful, suppressed, scanty, and irregular Menstruation, delayed development of puberty, &c. It is most suitable in delicate, atonic, extremely irritable persons, who are inclined to spasms, have a pale appearance, and disposed to leucorrhœa. DIERBACH advises it in spasms of the stomach and bowels, complicated with obstructions in the vena porta system, and irregularity of Menstruation. Labor-like pains in the uterus, with bearing-down and cutting pains, recurring at intervals—when menses set in 10 days too soon, but are scanty, lasting only 3 days.

Dose.—Same as for Chamomilla. (See page 43.)

ABSENT MENSTRUATION.

AMENORRHŒA.

In 1149 cases of uterine disease, ASHWELL met with 125 cases in which Menstruation was absent; in 181 other cases, MADDEN found 36 cases of the above disorder, *i. e.*, amenorrhœa, with 18 cases of irregular Menstruation, 35 cases of scanty discharge, 9 cases of late or delayed Menstruation, and 19 cases in which the flow was too pale in color.

A reference to the tables, (see pages 8 and 9,) will satisfy any one of the large number of cases which commence Menstruation at a late period, viz., after the 17th or 18th year. It is true, that in a large proportion of these cases, the patients suffered more or less in consequence of the delay. Under the gentle homœopathic treatment, there can be no objection in commencing the treatment of amenorrhœa as soon as the physician and mother have agreed that the proper time has arrived for the menstrual function to be established. If there be constitutional debility and delicacy of constitution to contend with, the treatment should be commenced very early, as these cases are always slower and more difficult of cure than are most other varieties of amenorrhœa; and, in the naturally delicate, if Menstruation does not quickly follow the advent of puberty, the patient generally suffers for months and years from the consequences of non-secretion; while COLOMBAT states, that under old school treatment, amenorrhœa, which has lasted several years, offers but slight chances of cure. The treatment in the dominant school is often so severe, that even the most experienced physicians prefer dilly-dallying with their cases in the commencement, and persist in their "masterly inactivity" until the disease becomes firmly established, and the general health of the patient is materially involved. Gentle treatment should be commenced with the first signs of declining health, and even before these appear, if the first advent of Menstruation be delayed beyond the 16th year. There are several varieties of Absent Menstruation, or amenorrhœa.

1. *When there is a slow and partial development, or entire absence of puberty.*

It is said that retarded Menstruation from absence of puberty, defective organization of the ovaries, or want of maturity in them, may be at once recognized by the general appearance of the girl; she is but a child, and has the appearance and manners of a child; and it is decidedly wrong to force or irritate the frail system of an immature creature. General invigorating management, however, should be instituted, the digestion improved, gymnastic exercises carefully followed up, fresh air, plain but generous diet, cheerful company, and agreeable variety of occupation and pleasure, should be supplied.

When there is a deficiency, or disorganization of the whole of both ovaries, the amenorrhœa will of course prove incurable; but as long as one, or even a portion of one ovary is sound, Menstruation may be performed more or less imperfectly; while partial, or remedial disease of the whole of both ovaries should be detected and removed. ASHWELL says, that when puberty and Menstruation are delayed from delicacy of constitution, or from residence in impure air, combined with sedentary employment, or when the general debility is owing to rapid growth of the whole body, thus diverting the requisite amount of nervous power and vascular activity from the ovaries and womb, that the majority of such cases will recover, under old school treatment, although months and years may elapse before the cure will be accomplished, during which time the confidence of the patient and of her friends, in medical skill, will be severely tested. In the N. A. Homœopathic Journal, Vol. 1, pp. 181 to 200, I have treated in full of *Atrophic ovarian*-amenorrhœa; Conium, Plumbum, Baryta, Muriatica, and Bromide of Potash, Camphora, Agnus castus, were there pointed out as the most homœopathic remedies to this condition; if these should fail, the Antipathic remedies, viz., Ferrum, Phosphor., Nux, Electricity, Stramonium, Aloes, and Cantharides, may be resorted to.

2. *Amenorrhœa after puberty is fully established.*

Retention of the menses beyond the period indicated naturally by the advanced development of the rest of the system, may arise

(a) From mere delicacy of the constitntion;

(b) From an irritable and hysterical condition;

(c) From chlorosis;

(d) From general plethora, especially when there is an excessively fibrinous state of the blood.

According to Ashwell and Loomis, who agree in a remarkable manner, not only in their views, but also in their language, amenorrhœa in plethoric, but otherwise healthy and robust subjects, is characterized by symptoms of congestion, or active plethora. There is headache, tension, and weight about the brain, with a sensation of fulness and throbbing in the centre of the head, or about the cerebellum, a florid countenance, torpor, lassitude, pain in the back and loins, a full, and generally a slow pulse, though occasionally, in irritable females, it is rapid; irregular circulation, evidenced by the feet and hands being, the one hot and the other cold, or both at short intervals remarkably hot or cold; the skin is sometimes harsh and dry, at others clammy. These symptoms at first pass away after the attempt at Menstruation is over, but subsequently they will persist during the intermenstrual periods, and recur in an aggravated degree as the menstrual epoch again approaches. This form is generally curable, though often neglected; and if long neglected, or inefficiently treated, a cure will not be soon accomplished.

The obstacles in the way of a cure by nature, or medical art, are:

1. An excess of blood in the whole system.
2. An excesssively fibrinous state of the blood.
3. Congestion of the womb so active, as to prevent the secretion of the menstrual fluid.

The principal homœopathic remedies for excess of blood in the whole system, are, Ferrum, China, Natrum muriaticum, Bellad., and Stramonium. The principal antipathic remedies, are, Aconite, Digitalis, Veratrum viride, Carbo vegetabilis and animalis.

The principal homœopathic remedy, against an excess of fibrin in the blood, is Argentum nitricum. The best antipathic remedies, are, Ferrum, Phosphor., Kali carb., Calcarea, Borax, Magnesia carb. and muriatica, Potassæ nitras, and Causticum.

The principal homœopathic remedies against congestion of the womb, are, Sabina, Stramonium, Cantharides, Aloes, Crocus, Platina, and the numerous remedies mentioned under the head of "Profuse Menstruation."

The varieties from debility and nervousness will be alluded to under the head of treatment.

3. *Amenorrhœa from distant disease, or visceral irritations, which retain the blood, and prevent it from being directed towards the womb.*

According to Colombat, amenorrhœa, depending upon disease of some organs, may set in at the commencement of such disease, or more frequently it appears at a rather advanced period; and it may be assumed as a general rule, that the menstrual derangement declares itself sooner in proportion to the degree of sympathy between the disordered organs and the womb; for example, when the stomach, brain, or heart is affected, the amenorrhœa is apt to come on at a very early period, whilst in consumption the complete suspension of the menses does not occur until the tubercles begin to soften. Very frequently the menstrual diarrhœa alluded to on page

14, becomes so prominent as to render the menses irregular, or even to suppress them; CHURCHILL has had patients, who, when their menses became irregular, were very liable to attacks of diarrhœa, with griping pain; BAUDELOCQUE knew a lady, 45 years old, who had never menstruated, but who had diarrhœa for 3 days in every month; BRERA, COLOMBAT, and FOUQUIER have seen cases in which dysentery sat in every month for several years, finally causing amenorrhœa. The simplest form of this variety of amenorrhœa occurs in consequence of the very rapid growth of the rest of the body, which diverts the nervous power and vascular activity from the ovaries and uterus, to the other and distant organs. COLOMBAT, in particular, insists that the menstrual flux may be prevented by all sorts of chronic, congestive, inflammatory, and nervous affections, and that very frequently a crowd of neuroses and neuralgias show themselves for the first time, only when Menstruation has become entirely suppressed, and yet they have caused the suppression, not merely arisen in consequence of it. With this clue we will be better able to understand the action of many remedies which have gained a reputation as emmenagogues, without exerting any specific action upon the ovaries or womb; they cure the distant irritations, and then merely allow the blood to return to its regular and periodical course; thus Bryonia will often remove chronic or periodical congestions to the chest, and afterwards allow the blood to be diverted downwards to the ovaries and womb; Bellad., by curing congestion to the head, homœopathically, will permit the regular menstrual congestion and hæmorrhage to take place from the womb; Veratrum, by allaying irritation of the bowels and curing diarrhœa, will remove the obstacle which prevented the blood from flowing towards the uterine organs.

Treatment.—In the Homœopathic Hospital Report, of 54 cases of suppressed, absent, or scanty Menstruation, 36 were cured, 7 relieved, and 11 uncured, or still under treatment. In the N. Y. Homœopathic Dispensary Report, for 1851, of 53 cases of suppressed or scanty Menstruation, 14 were cured, 34 relieved, and 5 unknown, or still under treatment. MAD-

DEN, in 94 cases of absent or scanty Menstruation, had 62 cases cured, or greatly benefitted; 27 cases somewhat benefitted; RÜCKERT reports 30 cases cured; BEAUVAIS, 24 cases; in all, 255 cases, of which 112 were cured or greatly benefitted; 68 somewhat relieved, and 43 uncured.

In RÜCKERT's Therapeutics, BEAUVAIS' and MALAIS' Cliniques, HENDERSON, &c., 65 cases of amenorrhœa cured by homœopathic remedies are reported: of these, 18 were cured by *Pulsatilla*, alone, and 12 by Pulsat., aided by other remedies; 8 cases were cured by *Sulphur*, alone, and 3 by Sulph., aided by other remedies; 6 cases were cured by *Nux vomica*, alone, and 4 cases by Nux, aided by other remedies; Sepia was used in 7 cases; Graphite was given in 10 cases; Calcarea in 5 cases; Bellad. in 3 cases; Aconite in 3 cases; Bryonia in 4 cases; Cocculus, Iodine, Opium, and Conium, each in 2 cases; Baryta, Caps., Stramon., Ant. crud., Natrum, Sabina, Coloc., Silex, Arnica, Ferrum, Carb. v., China, Urtica urens, and Nux moschata, each in 1 case.

PULSATILLA.

This is the favorite homœopathic remedy against amenorrhœa; we have already seen that it was given more or less successfully, in 26 cases out of 65. Hahnemann recommends it when the menses are suppressed or delayed, and attended with cramps in the bowels and womb. KNORRE found it useful when the patient's face was pale, and there was constant chilliness, even during summer weather and with warm clothing. TIETZE, when amenorrhœa was attended with leucorrhœa, dizziness, aching pain in the womb, and difficulty in urinating. KOPP, when there was great sensitiveness and weakness of the eyes. RÜCKERT, when there was menstrual colic, cutting pains in the bowels, pressure upon the bladder, attacks of vertigo, with loss of appetite and taste. TRINKS, in scanty Menstruation, when attended with menstrual colic. ALTSCHUL cured several cases with it. MADDEN found it very serviceable. But DIETZ and HEICHELHEIM, never witnessed any good effects from it, against absent Menstruation. An overdose of Pulsatilla is apt to cause pain in the stomach, canine hunger, nausea, and vomiting, slimy stools, frequent discharge of urine, profuse discharge of offensive sweat, excessive weakness, so that the patient is obliged to keep her bed, outbreak of a vesicular eruption over various parts of the body, trembling of the limbs, and peculiar pains in both eyes. VOGT says, that the most marked and constant of actions, are, increased flow of urine, and increased secretion of mucus from the nose and air tubes, and of perspiration. SOBERNHEIM says, that it acts upon the eyes and skin, mucous membranes, and urinary organs, in quite a specific manner. DIERBACH says, it causes offensive perspirations from the feet and arm pits, vesicular and pustular eruptions, profuse flow of urine, and that suppressed piles and menses are apt to reappear under its use; it is also apt to excite an irritation to cough, repeated sneezing, headache, dizziness, pain, sensitiveness, and dimness of the eyes, also nausea, vomiting, pains in the stomach and bowels, colic, and slimy diarrhœa. Hence, it would seem most homœopathic to amenorrhœa, and suppression from taking cold, especially if there be a catarrhal affection of the eyes, nose, and chest, or of the stomach and bowels; or a rheumatic catarrhal affection of these organs, and of the fibrous tissues. It is most homœopathic to amenorrhœa produced by visceral irritations in distant or gans, which retain the blood in the irritated parts, and prevent it from being directed towards the womb and ovaries. It is especially homœopathic to amenorrhœa from severe one-sided congestions to the head or eyes, or from severe scrofulo-catarrhal, or rheumatic inflammations of the eyes, nose, or lungs; from severe influenzas, chronic coryzas, or bronchitis; or from severe acute, or chronic mucous, or catarrhal irritations of the stomach and bowels, marked by slimy-coated tongue, nausea, loss of appetite, vomiting of mucus, pain in the stomach and bowels, and mucous diarrhœa; of from such severe catarrhal affection of the kidneys, bladder, uterus, and vagina, that the usual menstrual discharge is checked and prevented; finally, it is also homœopathic to amenorrhœa caused by skin diseases of great extent and tenacity, such as salt-rheum, acne, &c.

I have a strong suspicion, however, that it is antipathic to amenorrhœa, for STORK has seen it produce increased and copious Menstruation, and even flooding from the womb, attended with the discharge of thick, black blood; and DIERBACH says that suppressed piles and menses reappear under its use.

Dose.—The 2d dilution was used successfully in 1 case; the 4th in 3 cases; the 5th in 2 cases; the 6th in 3 cases; the 8th in 1 case; the 12th in 6 cases; and the 15th in 1 case. The very high dilutions do not seem to be thought worthy of confidence in this disease, as even Hahnemann advises 1 or 2 drop doses of the 12th dilution. TRINKS says, that the 2d dilution is by far the most useful, while ALTSCHUL prefers the 6th in adults. See also page 64.

GRAPHITE.

This remedy was used next most frequently to Pulsatilla, viz., in 10 cases. In my work on Headaches, page 110, I have pointed out the close relation of Graphite, or *mineral carbon*, to Sepia, or *fish carbon*, to Carbo vegetabilis, or *vegetable carbon*, and to Carbo animalis, or *animal carbon*. There is also a close relation between some of the actions of all these remedies, and those of Pulsatilla; at least they all act prominently upon the venous system and skin. Hahnemann found it most useful when there were frequent flushes of the face, troublesome dryness of the nose, eructations, morning-sickness, heaviness in the bowels, great accumulation of wind, obstinate constipation, painful piles, leucorrhœa, and coldness and falling asleep of the feet. TRINKS recommends it in scrofulous and venous constitutions, when there is a great inclination to perspire, and to chronic eruptions, or to catarrhal affections, or hæmorrhoidal and menstrual congestions to the upper part of the body. ALTSCHUL says, it is useful when catarrhal affections are apt to set in about the menstrual period, such as hoarseness, dry cough, evening-headache, and catarrhal fever, attended with pains in the bowels and small of the back, or by toothache, especially if diarrhœa occurs after the menstrual period has passed by. It has also been used successfully against suppressed, delayed, or irregular Menstruation, when there was a painful pressure upon the genital organs, persistent aching pains in the head, swelling of the belly and of the arms and legs, with heaviness and lassitude. Also, against amenorrhœa and dysmenorrhœa, from portal congestion; GOULLON used it successfully against amenorrhœa with dropsy of the feet; LOBETHAL against scanty and painful Menstruation, when the difficult irruption of the menstrual flow finally produces a scanty discharge, which generally soon ceases again. KNORRE recommends it from personal experience, against scanty and infrequent Menstruation, when it occurs irregularly, only every 8 or 10 weeks, and then lasts but a few days, with a scanty discharge of thick, black blood. LOOMIS recommends it when suppression occurs very soon after the flow commences, attended with cutting pains in the bowels, painful swelling in the region of the ovaries, a sensation as if everything was forced down towards the genital organs, headache, nausea, pains in the chest, a peculiar and characteristic white leucorrhœa, as liquid as water, especially if the patient be also troubled with herpetic or erysipelatous eruptions.

Dose.—The 12th dilution was used in 2 cases; the 30th in 5 cases. TRINKS recommends 1, 2, or 3 grain doses of the 1st, 2d, or 3d trituration; ALTSCHUL has seen excellent effects from the 2d dilution; LOBETHAL was very successful with the 1st and 2d potencies.

SEPIA.

This remedy is only reported as having been used in 7 cases, although it is given, perhaps, more frequently in *chronic* amenorrhœa, than any other homœopathic remedy. LOOMIS says, that it is appropriate in chronic amenorrhœa occurring in weakly females, with a delicate and tender skin, sallow complexion, and predisposition to melancholy and sadness, especially if they are also annoyed with a yellowish, or greenish-red, watery leucorrhœa, or a purulent, fetid, and corrosive discharge. Sepia-patients are subject to frequent attacks of nasal catarrh, suffer much with nervous debility, and tendency to weakening perspirations, with headache, nervous toothache, throbbing in the head, dizziness, bearing-down pain in the womb, pains in the loins and small of the back, and in the limbs, as if they had been bruised or beaten.

Tietze recommends it in those amenorrhœas which arise slowly out of an affection of the assimilation, and the whole bearing of the patient expresses the presence of an obstinate and deep-seated affection, the skin being pale, dingy, or sallow, the frame delicate, and the features marked with traces of frequent suffering. For Sepia to be useful, a dyscrasia should always be present, attended with obstinate and deep-seated nervous derangement. It is almost specific in cases attended with *sudor hystericus*, or a peculiarly sweetish-smelling perspiration of the arm-pits and soles of the feet.

Dose.—Same as recommended for Graphite.

SULPHUR.

This remedy was used more or less successfully in 11 cases. It is supposed to be a resolvent remedy which acts principally upon the skin, liver, mucous membranes of the bowels and lungs. It acts so beneficially upon the lungs and air tubes, that Graves always adds it to his cough prescriptions, and even in old times it obtained the name of "Balsam of the Lungs." Sundelin says, that it operates quite specifically upon the mucous membrane of the rectum, and thereby promotes critical hæmorrhoidal secretions; this action may be extended to the uterus, for Altschul says, that its exerts a specific influence upon the venous vessels of the abdomen, rectum, and pelvic organs; it causes congestion of blood to the womb, a pressing-down pain, and inflammation of the vulva, attended with too easy and too copious a flow of the menses, so that it probably cures amenorrhœa antipathically.

Loomis says, that it is most useful in the amenorrhœas of lymphatic and bilious females, predisposed to eruptions and enlargements of the glands; Knorre recommends it in suppressed Menstruation, when followed by congestion of blood to the head, especially when there is pain and heaviness in the occiput, extending down into the nape of the neck; also, when the patient's face is pale and sickly, with red spots or blotches upon the cheeks, and livid circles around the eyes; when the stomach is deranged, and there are sour eructations, with heaviness, fulness, pressure, and spasms in the stomach and bowels, loose and slimy stools, with straining, and inclination to piles; also, when there is pain in the loins, itching of the genital organs, and a yellowish, corrosive leucorrhœa. It is very useful when the suppression is preceded or followed by irritation or disease of the chest, marked by cough, more or less pain and soreness, shortness of breath, and expectoration of blood.

It is also particularly suitable in the amenorrhœas of bilious and rheumatic females, and when suppression is caused by a check of perspiration, from exposure to a current of air, or from getting wet, or washing in cold water.

Dose.—The tincture was used in 2 cases; the 1st trit. in 2; the 30th dilut. in 2; the 12th in 1 case. TRINKS recommends the 1st or 3d trituration, or 1 or 2 drop doses of the tincture. ALTSCHUL prefers the 1st or 6th dilution.

CALCAREA

Was given in 5 cases, although HAHNEMANN says it will never be given with benefit when there is a deficiency of the menstrual flow. It ought to prove far more homœopathic to amenorrhœa and diminished secretions from various parts, than either Pulsat., Graphite, Sepia, or Sulphur, for it not only diminishes the secretions of the gastro-intestinal mucous membrane, and thereby occcasions thirst and constipation, but with the exception of increasing the quantity of urine, when this is highly acid, it does not, like the other alkalies, promote the action of the different secreting organs, but rather diminishes it, and has, in consequence, been classed among the astringents.

It is thought to be most suitable for persons of a rickety, scrofulous, or lymphatic constitution, either with delicate frames from poor nutrition, or else with a great predisposition to grow large and fat. It will be treated of more fully under the head of chlorosis.

Dose.—HAHNEMANN found the 6th dilution most useful in robust persons. ALTSCHUL, who generally prefers the higher potencies, says that the latest experience of the best homœopathic physicians has proved, that the fear of the low dilutions is founded on imagination only. TRINKS prefers the 1st, 2d, or 3d trituration, or like dilutions of the *Spiritus Calcareæ.*

KALI CARBONICUM

Is frequently used by homœopathic physicians against amenorrhœa, although its principal action is to cause increased activity of the different secreting organs, and of the absorbing vessels and glands; it acts as a liquefacient and solvent, renders the blood thinner and darker colored, and causes it to lose its power of spontaneous coagulation when drawn from the body, and hence predisposes to hæmorrhage, and finally causes a state precisely similar to that of scurvy. It is one of the best antipathic remedies against that form of amenorrhœa which arises from an excessively fibrinous state of the blood, for it combines with fibrine and albumen, forming soluble compounds, or the so-called *fibrate and albuminate of potash;* gelatine is also readily dissolved by it. Dr. BLAUD, of Beaucaire, supposing that Ferrum does not exert all its curative properties, unless so modified as to be readily absorbed into the system, hit upon the plan of combining it with equal parts of the Kali sub. carbonicum, thinking thus to bring the Iron into a state of extreme division, rendering it more readily absorbed, while it acquires greater activity from its chemical combination. The great probability is, that the Kali modifies the blood, and diminishes the quantity of fibrin so much as to predispose the patient to hæmorrhage.

Dose.—Same as for Calcarea.

NUX VOMICA

Was used more or less successfully in 10 cases, although it has already been decided (see pages 28, 29, and 30) to be homœopathic to profuse Menstruation. It exerts a most powerful antagonistic action in debility of the nervous and muscular systems, and probably will relieve many cases of amenorrhœa attended with such defects. On the other hand, it, like Secale, is preëminently homœopathic to amenorrhœa from spasm, or tonic contraction and condensation of the womb, the muscular coat of this organ being so densely and rigidly contracted, that no secretion from it can take place. According to Loomis, it is useful when there is swelling of the womb, with great tenderness to touch, cramp-like and contracting pains, burning heat in the organ, and painful pressure towards the external parts. The action of Nux is very similar to that of Electricity. Strychnine, the active principle of Nux vomica, was first used as a remedy against amenorrhœa, by Dr. Bardsley, of Manchester; out of 12 cases, 10 were cured and 2 relieved. Churchill can add several cases in which the cure was permanent and complete. Although Bardsley's cases were of suppressed Menstruation, there is no reason for doubting its efficacy in simple amenorrhœa. Nauche has also used it successfully. Ashwell gave it in 4 cases, in delicate females, without success; Cholmeley used it in several instances unsuccessfully.

Dose.—Nux, 10th dilut., in one case restored the menstrual flow, after a cessation of 9 months; in 2 cases, the tincture was given every night and morning, at first 1 drop was given per dose, then the quantity was increased by 1 drop every day; the menses appeared on the 4th day in 1 case, on the 8th in the other. In most cases, the same doses as recommended for Ignatia, may be given. (See p. 57.)

ELECTRICITY.

To De Haen is supposed to belong the credit of first advocating the electric treatment of amenorrhœa, as early as 1758; he remarks that it always promotes the catamenial discharge. Birch, in 1779, published his Considerations on the Efficacy of Electricity in female obstructions, and from this time down to the present day, the value of this agent has been more or less recognised. Benert Bogin, was the first to use Galvanism in amenorrhœa; his first case was a girl, aged 18, and not yet regulated; she was galvinized 6 days, and on the

7th Menstruation sat in, and was soon followed by a perfect recovery of health. BOGIN cured several other cases. SCARPA also insisted particularly upon the emmenagogue properties of Electricity. ROGNETTA was not very successful with it, but found it more useful when applied to the hypogastrium and back, than when conveyed directly to the womb through the vagina. RAYER cured a suppression of several months' standing, at the 3d sitting. He also used Electricity in a female, subject to serious attacks of vomiting of blood, followed by amenorrhœa, which had been uselessly treated by various remedies, for 8 months; electro-magnetism was applied, once a day, for 10 or 15 minutes, strong enough to produce painless contractions; after the 5th sitting, the menses reappeared scantily, for 1 day only, but the vomiting of blood did not occur afterwards; Electricity was used again the next month, for several days previous to the expected period, and the menses then sat in more copiously, and the patient gradually recovered.

Lately, GOLDING BIRD has distinguished himself by his successful use of electricity in amenorrhœa; in 1843, he reported 24 cases treated by it; the youngest patient being 15 years old, the oldest 25, all unmarried.

Of these, 4 were chloretic,
6 slightly so,
12 not at all so,
2 complicated with hysteria.

Of these, the remedy succeeded in all except the four chlorotic girls.

BIRD says: "In electricity, we possess the only direct emmenagogue which the experience of our profession has furnished us with. I do not think I have ever known it fail to excite Menstruation where the womb was capable of performing this function. Disappointments, however, will almost certainly result at times, if we have recourse to electricity merely because a girl does not menstruate; and we must never lose sight of the fact, that, after all, the large majority of cases of amenorrhœa depend upon an anæmic, or bloodless condition of the patient, who does not menstruate simply because she has no blood to spare. Nothing can be more ridiculous than applying Electricity, or any other local irritant or stimulant, to the womb, when chlorosis exists; the first great indication will be to restore the general health; give Iron to make up for the previous deficiency of that element in the blood, [or give Kali carbonicum, or some other remedy, to reduce the excess of fibrin which prevents the hæmorrhage; or give Graphite, Sepia, or Sulphur, to remove the peculiar dyscrasias against which they are so specific; or use Nux vomica, to restore the tone of the digestive system, and remove excessive debility and irritability of the nervous and fibrous systems,] and then, and not before, think of stimulating the womb. It is true that, in a large proportion of cases, the menses will appear as soon as the chlorosis, [hyperinosis, dyscrasia, or general debility] is cured, and, of course, in such cases, there will be no need of the employment of Electricity; but still a large number will occur, in which, even after the complete relief of the chlorotic, anæmic [dyscratic, fibrinous, or debilitated] condition, the womb will remain torpid and refuse to act. In such cases, a few shocks of Electricity, transmitted through the pelvis, seldom, if ever, fail in effecting Menstruation. I have repeatedly known the menses, although previously absent for months, to appear almost immediately after the use of Electricity; and in more than one case the discharge actually appeared within a few minutes. About a dozen shocks should be transmitted through the pelvis, one director being placed over the lumbo-sacral region, the other just above the pubes, [or alternately over each ovarian region.]

Dr. McDonnell says, that the practitioner often meets with instances where females have suffered for months, or even years, from complete arrest of Menstruation, or from its being secreted scantily, and with difficulty and pain, or where the discharge comes on irregularly, being abundant and without pain at one time, whilst at the next period the patient may suffer exceedingly, scarcely any discharge being present; in another class of cases, severe dysmenorrhœa, or painful Menstruation may have existed for years before the physician is consulted. There are not, perhaps, any diseases in which the ordinary [allopathic] courses of treatment are more unsuccessful; for long before we are consulted, the usual effects of such derangements have become well marked upon the system; the constitution has become reduced and debilitated, and the ordinary features of chlorosis and hysteria have become well established. In other instances, the constitutional symptoms may have preceded the uterine derangements, and it often happens that the disease becomes more and more confirmed, and little or no benefit being derived from the advice of the regular [allopathic] physician, the patient resorts to quack medicines and nostrums, and after a waste of time, money, and health, a physician is again applied to. It is under such circumstances, and in such cases, that electro-galvanism acts with the greatest success, inducing a return of Menstruation when arrested, or producing an easy and abundant secretion, when the function has been scantily and painfully performed, perhaps for many years previously; and this change is soon followed by an amelioration of all the distressing symptoms under which the patient has labored.

McDonnell applies one button to the os pubis, the other is passed slowly along the spine, from the occiput to the os coccygis, four or five times, and then is kept applied to the sacrum for 5 or 6 minutes, and the Electricity is thus passed in an uninterrupted current through the uterus. It is by no means necessary to put the patient to great torture by increasing the strength of the shocks, as more benefit will be derived from an uninterrupted and steady transmission of a moderate quantity of electro-galvanism, than by occasional shocks of great intensity. The author reports several cases, which place the efficacy of electro-galvanism, in various uterine derangements, in a very favorable light.

The internal use of electrical remedies, such as Zinc and Cuprum, Zinc and Argentum, Zinc and Platina, 1 dose of each, to be given at an interval of ¼ or ½ hour, then allowing an intermission of 4 or 6 hours, and again repeating them in the same way, may be used with great benefit, in connection with the external application of Electricity.

SECALE

Acts specifically upon the nerves and muscles of the womb, almost in the same manner as Nux vomica and Electricity act upon the nerves and muscles in general. Although it is but rarely recommended in homœopathic works, it ought to prove one of the very best homœopathic remedies against painful, scanty, and suppressed Menstruation. It has been frequently used in the old school, notwithstanding its homœopathicity; CHURCHILL says: that Ergot of Rye will increase, if not originate, uterine contractions, is known to all, and also, that it will restrain inordinate discharges from the womb; we should, however, scarcely expect it to be useful in exciting the menstrual secretion, and it is difficult [easy] to determine upon what principle it does so. As to the fact, we have the evidence of DEWEES, who recommends its use; of Dr. LOCOCK, who has tried it with success; and of ROCHE, NAUCHE, and PAULY.

Dose.—In scanty or suppressed Menstruation, Secale should be given in quite small, or homœopathic doses; it often fails in the hands of old school physicians, because they administer it in 5 or 10 grain doses, several times a day. In *profuse* Menstruation, however, in which it is antipathic, it should be given in full doses. I have been to the habit of relying upon it, almost exclusively, in menorrhagia, and have rarely or never known it to fail. In suppressed or scanty Menstruation, the 1st, 2d, or 3d dilution may be given once or twice a day, during the interval, and every 4, 6, or 8 hours, during the menstrual period. Or, from 2 to 4 granules may be administered as often as above directed.

BRYONIA

Was used in 4 cases, although it has already been decided to be homœopathic to profuse and frequent Menstruation. (See pages 28, 29, and 40.) It is probably homœopathic to amenorrhœa, when the menses are delayed or suppressed by the counter-irritant action of rheumatism of the chest, joints, or limbs; and homœopathic to profuse Menstruation from rheumatism of the womb or ovaries.

Dose.—See pages 40 and 41.

BELLADONNA

Was used in 3 cases, although it also has been said to be homœopathic to profuse Menstruation. See page 39.

Dose.—See pages 39 and 40.

ACONITE

Was also used in 3 cases; it, too, has been recommended as an emmenagogue. See page 36.

Dose.—See page 36.

OPIUM

Was only used in 2 cases, although it is decidedly one of the most homœopathic remedies to scanty, suppressed, or absent Menstruation, although PEREIRA says that the menses, lochia, and secretion of milk, are not checked by it, and that its use in the female is not likely to be attended with suppression or retention of the uterine or mammary secretions. It is most homœopathic when amenorrhœa is attended with congestion of blood to the head, obstinate constipation, and scanty urine.

Dose.—Same as for Aconite.

CONIUM

Is also one of the most undoubted homœopathic remedies for amenorrhœa. DIERBACH says, that it exerts an especially depressing action upon the genital organs, preventing pollutions, relieving satyriasis and nymphomania, and repressing ordinary sexual inclination to such a degree, that in olden times the Hierophantes and priests of Cybele, were obliged to use Conium juice internally, and also to wash themselves with it, in order to keep down all lustful emotions. ANDRY, ANDREE, and GREDING, assert that it causes suppression; LIN-

NÆUS knew it to cause impotence in one instance; HAHNEMANN says, that it causes suppression of the menses, with pains in the back and sacrum, also scanty menstrual flow, and barrenness. It also exerts an equally depressing effect upon the breasts and testicles, to that which it induces in the womb and ovaries; DOSCORIDES says, it suppresses the milk in women, and prevents the development of the breasts in virgins, and causes a wasting away of the testes in boys. PLINY gives a similar account of its action, and says that it reduces all tumors. AVICENNA praises it as a remedy for tumors of the breasts and testicles, while, more recently, PEREIRA has heard of 2 cases in which it caused atrophy of the female breasts. It is homœopathic to amenorrhœa from atrophy and torpor of the ovaries and womb.

Dose.—Same as for Belladonna.

BARYTA

Was used in 1 case only, although it is almost as homœopathic to amenorrhœa, as Secale or Conium; it produces atrophy of the womb, ovaries, and breasts, and diminishes the sexual feeling more decidedly than any other remedy.

Dose.—Same as for Calcarea. See page 48.

KREOSOTE.

My friend, Dr. BOLLES, cured 1 case of amenorrhœa, of 1 years' standing, with Kreosote 30.

EMMENAGOGUES.

In those cases of amenorrhœa in which strictly homœopathic remedies fail to effect a cure, or else, as they frequently do, restore the general health without bringing on the menstrual flow, it may be allowable to use moderate doses of emmenagogue remedies. If WHITEHEAD'S opinion is correct, that Menstruation is merely a flow of blood from the womb and its appendages, and not a peculiar secretion, then there are many remedies well calculated to favor the excretion. Of these:

SABINA

Is the most certain and powerful. (See page 65.)

Stramonium, Ferrum, Aloes, Cantharides, Crocus, Borax, Ruta, Nux vomica, Potash, and others, are well-tried and efficient remedies. As the same blood vessels and nerves furnish branches to the bladder, kidneys, womb, ovaries, and rectum, some German physicians have hit upon the idea of giving Aloes, which acts specifically upon the rectum; Sabina, which operates especially upon the womb; and Cantharides, which effects the bladder so decidedly, in order to draw down the blood from the upper parts of the body, to all of the pelvic viscera. But this treatment will fail entirely, unless anæmia has been previously removed by the use of Ferrum or Manganum; excess of fibrin by means of Kali carb., Kali nit.; deficiency of nervous energy, by Phospor. or Nux; deep-seated dyscrasias, by Sepia, Graphite, Carbo animalis, etc.

In some cases all these remedies will fail, and even the most bigotted theoretical physician will at times be glad to resort to some empirical remedy.

PRUNUS LAUROCERASUS.

Dr. Kastner, first tried the efficacy of this drug upon a strong, plethoric girl, aged 16, in whom the symptoms of Menstruation had appeared a year before, but latterly had almost entirely ceased. She suffered at times, however, with considerable distress, such as congestion to the head and chest, and also violent colics; these symptoms becoming much increased, Dr. K. tried many of the usual remedies, but without effect; he at length became acquainted with the use of this bark, and 6 days before the next periodic return of the symptoms, she was ordered to use it daily. On the expected day the usual disagreeable symptoms came on, viz., loss of appetite, rumbling in the bowels, frequent desire to pass water, with a burning sensation during micturition, dragging sensation in the pelvis, with rush of blood to the head; two days thereafter a mucous discharge appeared from the vagina, and on the third day a diarrhœa, along with the menstrual flow, which continued moderately for 4 days. The next period was 2 days too late, and the next again 3 days too early, but after this she became quite regular.

Two other similar cases were treated with an equally favorable issue; and lastly, a case of suppression, in a girl, aged 18, in whom, after using the medicine for two separate periods of 8 days each, the discharge was reëstablished.

CHENOPODIUM OLIDUM.

Dr. Holton has had frequent opportunities of watching the curative action of this remedy, and is perfectly convinced that it is a very safe and important medicine in many cases in which Menstruation is not duly performed; he generally gave it for a fortnight previous to the expected menstrual period, and repeats the same treatment if the first course of it does not effect a cure. It will cure cases in which restoration of the general health is not followed by Menstruation, and the womb itself requires assistance.

MAMMARY IRRITATION.

Dr. Cormack says, that warmth und stimulants applied to the breasts often act powerfully as emmenagogues; in the ordinary treatment of amenorrhœa, the first indications of the womb being roused from its torpor are turgescence and tingling of the breasts; phenomena which also usually precede natural Menstruation. It is equally true, though not so familiarly understood, that measures which act directly and primarily upon the breasts, such as warm clothing to the breasts, and the application of ordinary or stimulating poultices, not only cause them to swell and throb, but likewise stimulate the ovaries and cause the menses to flow. The practice of applying leeches to the breats in amenorrhœa, owes its efficacy to the fomentations used, and the irritation of the bites.

Drs. Cormack and Patterson give 1 case, in a woman, aged

24, in whom the menses had been suppressed for 2½ years, cured in 2 days by the application of a large mustard poultice to one breast. Also, another case, in a girl, aged 19, with suppression for 5 months, cured in 3 days by a mustard poultice to one half of one breast.

The emmenagogue effects ascribed to the application of the leaves of the Castor oil plant, by Drs. McNilham and Tyler Smith, can easily be understood, when we remember their irritating character, and the consequences which have been found to follow irritation of the breasts by other stimulants. A good deal may be effected by the mere application of warm poultices.

SUPPRESSED MENSTRUATION.

Two great varieties are generally admitted, viz., *Sudden* or *Acute* suppression, and *Gradual* or *Chronic*;—*temporary* suppression also deserves attention.

Sometimes the suppression is very simple and temporary in its nature, and merely requires time to remove it. Tilt says, that mothers should be made aware of the fact, that without any detriment to a girl's health, Menstruation may be suppressed by any great change of abode, or circumstances; that when a girl leaves the country and goes to school in town, the flow will be very likely to stop for 3 or 6 months, and then proceed regularly, even without medical treatment; and *vice versa*, when a girl is accustomed to a town residence, she will be apt to have a cessation for a short time, if she passes the summer in the country, although the suppression may not come on until she returns to the city again.

Tilt says that this fact is so little known by women, that he was scarcely surprised at being informed by Dr. Julius, of Richmond, that in a school which he attended professionally, where the number of boarders generally averaged from 80 to 90 girls, this *retard* or delay in the regular appearance of Menstruation, occurred so frequently soon after the arrival of the girls, that the lady presiding over the establishment, felt convinced that it depended on the unwholesomeness of the situation, and she intended to urge the removal of the institution to another locality, had not Dr. JULIUS succeeded, with some difficulty, in convincing her of the real state of the case.

That this *temporary suppression* depends on change only, and not on a change from agreeable to less agreeable circumstances, is proved by the fact, that when the courses have proceeded regularly in town, they sometimes stop for several months when a girl returns to her home in the country.—TILT. The suppression probably depends upon the same causes which so frequently induce obstinate constipation, when a change from city to country, or *vice versa*, has been made, coupled with a more or less great change in diet, water, hours of eating, &c., all aided by the powerful excitement to the brain and nervous system, induced by the novelty of the new mode of life. This view is corroborated by the similar effects of a sea voyage, especially upon those who are not familiar with the beauties and terrors of the sea, and are unaccustomed to the motion of a vessel. Menstruation is almost always arrested and suppressed during a sea voyage, and seldom recommences until several months after an arrival in a strange land. This is observed to take place as frequently with ladies arriving in India, after a long sea voyage, as it is with the poor Irish emigrant to America.

COLOMBAT asserts, that suppression, which occurs in the year following the first appearance of the menses, is rarely of much importance, as it is scarcely ever due to a seriously morbid state of the womb. TILT has noticed that those girls who attain to puberty very early, are seldom quite regular before the age of 18, and says, if these facts were to be carefully instilled into the mother's mind, there would be much less mischief done by the injudicious administration of forcing medicines to promote the return of what, in fact, ought not to have appeared so soon.

Suppressed Menstruation may be produced by *moral*, *physical*, *unknown* causes, or by those symptomatic of some disorder of distant organs, or acute irritation of any part of the body.

Brierre de Boismont, in 190 cases of suppression, found it produced by

Moral causes in . . .	92	instances.
Physical " . . .	68	"
Unkown " . . .	30	"
	190	

Among the *moral* causes may be mentioned anger, disappointed love, jealousy, excessive joy, sudden reception of bad news, fright, extreme fear, or sudden disappointment. From the report of Baudelocque, we learn that 62 women were attacked with hæmorrhage or suppressions on the occasion of the explosion of the powder magazine of Grenelle; Husson witnessed a case in which menstrual suppression had been caused at several different times by the mental shock, at hearing loud claps of thunder; Colombat observed in July, 1830, that the report arising from the platoon-firing and cannon shot, produced the same effect on several women; Rostan had a patient whose "monthlies" became suddenly suppressed on learning that a seton was to be applied to her chest; one of Colombat's relatives, whose Menstruation was ordinarily very regular and abundant, was attacked with sudden suppression, in consequence of a frightful dream and kind of night-mare; Churchill says, that almost all the women who are sent up to the Richmond Penitentiary, labor under suppression of the menses, in consequence of the mental agitation and distress they have undergone; Gooch relates, that a patient of his consulted him long after the entry of the Cossacks into Paris, for suppression, which was solely produced by the alarm she then suffered. The influence of the brain and nervous system in producing suppression, is perhaps more generally acknowledged, and more adroitly treated by homœopathic physicians than by any others; they regard it as far more important to allay the derangement of the nervous system, and then to allow the blood and vital energies to be directed to their proper channels by nature, than to attempt to force Menstruation.

Aconite, Lycopod., Kali c., Coffea, Opium, or Veratrum, will be suitable when suppression is caused by fright, or sudden mental emotion.

Acon., Bell., Coloc., Ignatia, Platina, Puls., or Staph., are recommended when it is caused by mortification of mind, or contradiction.

Bryonia, Cham., or Colocynth, when caused by a fit of passion.

Coffea, or Opium, if by excessive joy.

Ignatia, Hyos., Phos. ac., or Hellebore, if produced by disappointed love, etc.

Among the *physical* causes of suppression, the application of cold is the most common and dangerous; such as sudden exposure to cold and damp air, immersion of the feet and hands in cold water, cold hip-baths, sitting upon the grass, or ground, use of ice cream or very cold drinks, when the body is over-heated, or the leaving off of an accustomed garment; PULTE says, that he has foundthe wearing of thin-soled shoes to be the most fruitful source of the decay of female beauty, and the decline of female health; the injury of tight lacing, although considerable, is nothing in comparison with the fatal habit of appearing in all kinds of weather in thin-soled shoes and gossamer stockings. There is a very large class of young girls who are apt to have "a check" from the slightest chill or exposure during the monthly period, yet they will obstinately persist in trudging out in snow or rain storms, to church, or school, or to places of amusement, or will loiter in cold rooms while dressing or undressing, or will walk about in their bare or stocking feet, etc. Happily or unhappily, the effect of several of these causes may be diminished by the frequency of their occurrence, so that bathing women go into the sea, during Menstruation, with perfect impunity, and the habitual exposure to the casualties of life, necessarily diminishes their injurious impression. It would be a useless task for a physician to attempt to reform the evening dresses of ladies; TILT truly says, that rich young ladies suffer as much from insufficient clothing as the daughters of the destitute; for poverty and fashion are two inexorable tyrants, which exact the same things and often bring on the same diseases; enough has been said against the exposure of the upper part of the chest, and the "diaphanous attire" of young ladies; they at least do not yet fully rival the belles of Axim, on the coast of Africa, it being a positive fact, that some of the Axim girls wear merely the bustle, without so much as the shadow of a garment. The Axim mothers, however, have a reason for wearing a *tournure* which does not exist elsewhere, for their little children ride astride of the maternal "tarb Roshe," which thus becomes useful, as well as ornamental.—BRIDGE.

Among other physical causes of suppression may be mentioned, the use of purgatives or emetics about the time of Menstruation, large doses of chincona, the action of strong odors, particularly, according to HALLER's assertion, of the herb Pennyroyal; DE BOISMONT says, that Copaiba and Cubebs are very apt to produce amenorrhœa; Opium, Plumbum, and Secale, would be likely to produce the same effects, also many of the styptic remedies, and those employed in the old school against menorrhagia.

According to ASHWELL, sudden suppression in stout, plethoric, and ruddy females, will be followed by active congestion, if not by inflammation; the patient immediately feels a sensation of heat, weight, and pain in the pelvis, more or less violent uterine colic, and a disagreeable fulness and tension in the groins, and loins, and upper part of the thighs; the abdomen and breasts become enlarged; there is an indescribable feeling of *malaise* and lassitude; extreme loathing, nausea, vomiting, headache, dizziness, noises in the ears, oppression of the chest, frequent palpitations, and in many, a burning pain while urinating. Suppression, accompanied by such symptoms, is far more immediately dangerous than any of the other derangements of Menstruation.

Treatment.—LOOMIS recommends Aconite when the pulse is rapid, or full and sluggish; a rush of blood to the head, producing pain; giddiness and drowsiness, with flushing of the face; weight in the loins, especially if there be heat, thirst, and a general feverish state.

Dose.—See page 36.

BELLADONNA

May be given, if the head be hot, the face alternately pale or flushed, the limbs cold, and there be shiverings alternating with heat, and attended with confusion of the head; or if there be dizziness, trembling of the hands, sparkling before the eyes, with aching pains in the eyeballs and sockets; shooting pains about the womb and ovaries, with heat and dryness of the vagina.

Dose.—See page 40.

BRYONIA

Is recommended when there is congestion to the head or chest, with vertigo, bleeding of the nose, stitches in the sides of the chest, and dry cough, attended with constipation, severe pressing pain in the stomach, or by colic and irritability of temper.

Dose.—See page 40.

NUX VOMICA

May be given, when there is swelling of the womb, with great tenderness to touch, cramp-like and spasmodic pains in the womb, with burning heat in, and painful pressure towards, the external parts.

Dose.—Same as Ignatia. (See page 57.)

OPIUM

May be useful in recent cases, when there is great heaviness of the head, dizziness, lethargy, and drowsiness, or excessive desire to sleep without the ability to accomplish it, the pulse being full and slow; especially if there also be obstinate constipation, and retention of urine.

Dose.—Same as Crocus. (See page 55.)

When suppression occurs in delicate and spare women, who are highly nervous and irritable, inflammation may occur; but in the majority of such attacks, the pain and other symptoms are not inflammatory, although it is sometimes difficult to distinguish the aggravated neuralgia and spasm of the different abdominal organs, and of the womb and its appendages, from real inflammation. In these cases, the pain is rarely fixed, but attacks first one organ, then another, changing its locality without the use of remedies; it is often remarkable, how quickly the pain may be transferred from the womb to the head, from the head to the chest or heart, or again from these parts to the bowels; the patient is also apt to have hysteric, or fainting fits.

Treatment.—*Pulsatilla* may be given when the prominent symptoms are languor, pain across the small of the back and lower part of the bowels, palpitation, nausea, vomiting, sensation of fulness in the head and eyes, and disposition to general coldness, especially if there be alternate crying and laughter, or sadness and melancholy; the pains being particularly inclined to shift their location rapidly and repeatedly.

Dose.—See pages 64 and 95.

COCCULUS

Is indicated, when there is great derangement of the nervous system, violent cramps in the bowels, and womb, the patient being very weak, and agitated, with sighing and moaning.

Dose.—Same as Ignatia. (See page 57.)

VERATRUM

Is indicated, if the suppression be the result of fear, fright, or vexation, attended with, or followed by anger, especially if hysterical affections set in, or nervous headache, the face being pale and earthy, the hands, feet, and face cold, followed by extreme debility and fainting, or nausea and vomiting, with acidity, or by diarrhœa.

Dose.- Same as Bryonia. (See page 41.)

NUX MOSCHATA

Is said to be adapted to acute suppression, when caused by a chill from being in the water, or exposure to cold and damp air, especially when it occurs in persons of a nervous and mobile constitution, and is attended with spasms or other nervous affections, or by great drowsiness, or inclination to faint, with sense of great fatigue and exhaustion, and pain in the loins.

Dose.—Same as Chamomilla. (See page 43.)

CUPRUM

Is indicated when there is a pressing pain on the top of the head, rush of blood to the head and face, with redness of the face and eyes, or else paleness of the face with livid circles around the eyes, nausea and vomiting, cramps of the stomach and bowels, convulsive movements of the limbs, spasms of the chest, and palpitation of the heart.

Dose.—Same as Ignatia. (See page 57.)

CHRONIC SUPPRESSION.

This disease will be treated of fully under the head of Amenorrhœa, or absent Menstruation.

VICARIOUS MENSTRUATION.

Colombat says, among the most curious phenomena following suppression of the menses, should be ranked the hæmorrhages and other vicarious discharges. They take place more frequently from the mucous membranes, especially of the lungs, stomach, and bowels, than from other parts, although they have been met with from almost every region of the body. Thus, Gardien observed a girl who, after suppression of Menstruation, had a periodical discharge of blood: 1st, for 6 months from small ulcers on the legs; 2d, for a year, from ulcers upon the arms; 3d, for 6 months, from the opening of a felon on the left thumb; 4th, for 2 years, from ulcers at the angle of the eye, in consequence of erysipelas of the face; 5th, for 5 months, from the navel, where another erysipelas had made its appearance; 6th, for 4 months from the inner side of the left ancle; 7th, and finally, for 2 months, from the left ear. In this case, when the blood ceased to flow from a given point, the patient was seized with attacks of bleeding from the nose or lungs, preceded by convulsions, headache, and dizziness.

Dr. Chatelain had a patient, who, in consequence of derangement of Menstruation, had discharges of blood successively from the arm-pit, nipple, left flank, back, pit of the stomach, and the thigh.

Begin had a young person, whose fore-finger of the left hand, swelled, and was covered with an acute herpetic eruption, from the surface of which blood flowed at a certain period every month. The eruption and the discharge, which only lasted 3 or 4 days each time, were accompanied by a disagreeable itching. Three years after, the womb returned to its natural functions, and the health of the patient was reëstablished.

Rousseau states, that a woman had suppression in consequence of the shock from the extraction of a molar tooth, and a discharge, which was renewed every month, was established from the socket of this tooth. Raymond, also, speaks of a woman who had a bleeding once a month from the socket of a tooth which she had lost; the discharge of blood, which lasted 3 days, amounted to 3 ounces per day, or 9 ounces per term. Pechlin had a case of vicarious Menstruation from an ulcer on the foot; Kerckring cites the case of a girl who was periodically regulated from a wound in the right hand. Mercatus had a woman with suppression, whose cheeks became of a very deep red color every month. —Colombat.

Leadam had a young lady under his care, who was subject to oozing of blood from the upper surface of all the toes, a few days before Menstruation, which was always scanty. Also, a young married woman, who had never been pregnant, and whose Menstruation was very irregular, who, every 3 or 5 weeks, first had serum, then blood, ooze out of the right nipple. And a third patient, with attacks of bleeding of the lungs for a year or two, with suppression of the menses, who had, before the occurrence of the blood-spitting, an oozing of blood from the scalp, just above the forehead; this was repeated 2 or 3 times, and so alarmed her friends, that they ran off with her to a physician, with the blood trickling down her forehead.

The general impression of the profession seems to be, that no serious results follow these bleedings, even when delicate organs are the seat of it; on the contrary, they are said to prevent in a great measure the occurrence of those severe and fatal diseases, which sometimes follow upon amenorrhœa. Sooner or later, the womb resumes its functions, and this disagreeable succedaneum subsides.

LOOMIS, with mingled gravity and modesty, asks what are the causes of this disorder? He says, suppression of Menstruation cannot be the cause, because suppression is not always followed by Vicarious Menstruation. He, again, boldly assumes, that plethora or congestion cannot be the cause, because these are met with in thousands of cases, without any vicarious discharge. And finally concludes, that it is better to say that we "do not know the why"!! But, as Menstruation is a simple but periodical hæmorrhage from the womb, it is not at all strange, when it is suppressed, that we should meet with periodical discharges from any part more irritated than the uterus. Thus, according to STAHL, an indigestion or pulmonary catarrh, occurring during Menstruation, will suffice to provoke the flow of blood towards the stomach or lungs. We also find that bleeding from the nose, stomach, lungs, and bladder, are the most common forms of vicarious hæmorrhage, just as they are the most frequent varieties of accidental hæmorrhage. Again, in young females, the vicarious bleeding generally takes place from the nose, stomach, or chest; later in life, the hæmorrhoidal vessels and bladder are apt to be the seat of the flux. We have already seen (see page 91,) that irritations of distant organs invite and provoke the flow of blood from the womb to the irritated part, and thus frequently cause suppression; the irritation may be great enough to produce a discharge of blood; and, finally, the periodicity of Menstruation will impress a periodical character upon the vicarious bleedings, in the same way that it impresses a regular type upon the headaches, colics, and what not, which so frequently attend Menstruation.

Treatment.—LEADAM recommends *Ferrum* as the homœopathic remedy for most of these cases; Millefolium may often prove useful. He cured one case of vicarious bleeding from the nipple, with Lycopodium.

LOOMIS suggests Ferrum, Mur., Lachesis, and Lycopod., when the bleeding is from the *skin.*

If from the nose, Bryon., Puls., Sepia.

If from the eyes, Bell., Carb. v., Cham., or Nux vom.

If from the ears, Bryon., Cicuta, Graph., Merc., Petrol., Puls., Rhus.

If from the mouth and gums, Arnica, Bell., Cham., Ferrum mur., Kreosot, Ledum, and Lycopodium.

If from the lungs, he suggests 30 remedies, all of which have some little reputation against simple bleeding from the lungs.

If from the stomach, one or the other of 16 remedies, which are commonly recommended for Hæmatemesis.

If from the bladder, 14 of the most common remedies for hæmaturia.

CHLOROSIS.

GREEN SICKNESS.

Several entirely different disorders may be combined with and mistaken for simple chlorosis, viz.:

1st. Anæmia, or deficiency of blood;

2d. Hydræmia, or watery condition of the blood;

3d. Leucocythemia, or excess of white cells in the blood.—Bennett.

It is exceedingly difficult to separate chlorosis distinctly from these other affections; in fact, as already stated, several of them often occur in varying degrees of combination.

In 1149 cases of uterine disease, Ashwell met with 89 examples of chlorosis, and Tilt asserts that the frequency of chlorosis is greater than is generally believed; for although physicians are only consulted for it in extreme cases, two-thirds of all women residing in large towns are more or less tinged with this complaint.

According to Colombat, no disease inspires more tender interest, or more touching compassion, than the state of paleness, suffering, and languor, observed in a young chlorotic girl; like some delicate plant deprived of the beneficent rays of the sun, she is a flower which withers and droops away, even before its blossoming.

The approach of chlorosis is marked by a state of habitual inertia and melancholy (Ignatia); the patient becomes sombre and taciturn, weeps without cause, and sighs involuntarily (Puls., Aurum); the face may become bloated, and the expression, as it were, veiled (Arsen. Plumbum); the eyes are sad and languishing; the eyelids, which may be swollen, especially in the morning, are encircled by blackish rings, contrasting strongly with the pearly color of the whites of the eyes, and the pallor of the lips; the skin, particularly of the extremities, is dry and cool; the pulse frequent, rather large, and easily compressed; the breathing difficult; digestion deranged; the alvine dejections become white and hard (Plumbum), but sometimes are fluid; palpitations, and creeping chilly turns, make their appearance, while debility, lassitude, a desire for sleep, or rather for repose, augment from day to day.—Colombat.

The patient feels a frequent inclination to make deep and very strong inspirations, which is increased by walking, ascending, or even by very slight exercise, and finally, by any mental emotion; the impulse of the heart is stronger, and the carotid arteries, which beat with great force, are the seat of certain peculiar and unnatural sounds. Sometimes we have the simple or double bellows sound; at others, a prolonged vibration, and a kind of humming, like that produced by a humming-top.

As the disease progresses, the functions of the stomach become deranged; the strangest and most depraved appetites may manifest themselves, and it is not uncommen for chlorotic patients to prefer the most sapid substances, such as salt, vinegar, or green fruits, while they often seek with avidity indigestible substances, such as charcoal, chalk, plaster, earth, ashes, spiders, flies, and other equally disgusting objects. The appetite may gradually diminish, or be increased beyond measure, while the ingestion of food is followed by a sense of weight at the pit of the stomach, and sometimes by vomiting. The tongue is generally large, and covered with a mucous coat; acid regurgitations, and frequent nausea, occur, especially in the morning; a feeling of heat and weight in the pit of the stomach, and sometimes nervous pains in the course of the gullet, and extending through to the shoulders, make their appearance. Finally, the patients experience alternations of constipation and watery diarrhœa, the passages being white, while the urine is small in quantity, pale, and limpid, as in by many nervous affections.—COLOMBAT.

The nervous system participates in the general languor of all the functions; the patient becomes sad, melancholic, and indifferent to all enjoyment; she seeks solitude, sighs involuntarily, and weeps without cause; she is often tormented with sinister ideas; her temper is capricious, odd, and irascible; for her, all thought and hope of happiness is gone, and in her despair she often speaks of suicide; her nights are disturbed broken slumbers and frightful dreams.—COLOMBAT.

Various nervous symptoms may be added, such as noises in the ears, dizziness, partial loss of sight, tremors of the limbs, neuralgic pains in the head, neck, or teeth, peculiar palpitations in the pit of the stomach, and hysterical symptoms. When the progress of the disease is not arrested, the symptoms become more and more aggravated; the head becomes the seat of severe pain, felt especially in the back of it; the skin assumes a greenish or earthy hue; the stomach and bowels become hard and tumid, thirst sets in; the difficulty of breathing, faintness, and palpitations, are increased; diarrhœa and hectic fever gradually creep in; daily aggravations occur, and emaciation makes rapid progress. Finally, the presence of slight general dropsy, extreme debility, invincible repugnance to all kinds of exertion, marked alteration of the features, and a pale violet color of the lips, forebode approaching death, which comes at last without shock and without pain.

The disease is supposed to depend upon one or more of three or four causes, viz:

1st. Debility of the digestive organs.

2d. Weakness of the genital organs, with amenorrhœa from debility.

3d. Debility of the circulatory system, with a depraved state of the blood.

4th. General debility of the nervous system, especially of the nerves which preside over the circulation, digestion, nutrition, and genital functions.

Colombat decides that atony of the digestive organs ought not to be considered as the starting-point of the disease, as chlorosis sometimes precedes the derangement of the digestive organs, and even the stomach at times retains its natural condition. He also asserts, that debility of the ovaries and womb, with absence of Menstruation, cannot be regarded as the primary cause of the chlorotic condition, for this sometimes makes its appearance in well-regulated girls, who do not cease to be so throughout the disease; it has also been observed in women who menstruate abundantly and perfectly, and in pregnant females. But it is very true, that a profuse leucorrhœal discharge often takes the place of Menstruation; that the menses generally fail, or become suppressed; and even when they persist and last longer than usual, the excreted fluid is apt to be pale and watery, to separate upon the napkin into two distinct portions, and form spots which lose all their color by drying. He also rejects the theory which supposes the chlorotic condition to depend upon debility of the blood and blood-vessels, producing a depraved state of the composition of the blood, marked by *excess* of serum, and of the white particles of the blood, including the fibrin, and a *deficiency* of coloring matter, blood globules, Iron, and even of Manganese, which latter is now regarded as a natural and invariable ingredient of the blood. However this may be, the alterations in the composition of the blood are among the earliest and most characteristic features of the disease. Thus, in 8 cases of slight chlorosis, observed by ANDRAL, the water of the blood was *increased* from the natural standard of $\frac{790}{1000}$ to $\frac{801}{1000}$; while in 18 confirmed cases of the disease, the water was increased to $\frac{853}{1000}$, and in a few cases even to $\frac{870}{1000}$, giving rise to a serous plethora of great importance, *i. e.*, to the so-called *Hyperhydræmia*, which is attended with signs of blood-fulness, and turgor lymphaticus, the blood actually being in excessive quantity, although it is watery, pale, and thin.

Again, the natural quantity of fibrin in healthy blood, is 3 parts in 1000, while in chorosis it often rises to $\frac{3.609}{1000}$ or to $\frac{3.5}{1000}$, and even to $\frac{5.3}{1000}$, and as the coagulability of the blood depends in a great measure upon the quantity and quality of the contained fibrin, we can readily see that hæmorrhage will not be apt to take place in chlorosis.

The coloring matter and blood globules are greatly *diminished;* in ANDRAL's 8 cases of slight chlorosis, the blood globules were diminished from the natural standard of $\frac{127}{1000}$ to $\frac{106}{1000}$, while in the 18 severe and confirmed cases, they were further lessened to an average of $\frac{60}{1000}$, and in exceptional cases they were decreased to $\frac{40}{1000}$, and even to $\frac{30}{1000}$, forming a class of clases in which the amount of blood globules fell so far below the natural standard, that we can scarcely comprehend how life could still have been maintained.

Finally, according to LECANU, from $\frac{8}{1000}$ to $\frac{6}{1000}$ of Iron are found in the blood of healthy females, while only from $\frac{3}{1000}$ to $\frac{5}{1000}$ are present in that of chlorotic persons.

The quantity of Manganese in the blood in health and in this disease has not yet been determined.

This will, perhaps, be the most proper place to point out the difference between Anæmia, Hydræmia, and Leucocythemia.

ANÆMIA.

Deficiency of Blood.

The analogy between anæmia and chlorosis is so great, that ANDRAL regards them as one and the same disease. Among the symptoms common to both, are: paleness and discoloration of the skin, whites of the eyes, lips, and mucous membrane of the mouth; shrinking and disappearance of the subcutaneous veins; muscular debility; fainting from the slightest exertion; dropsical swellings; derangement of the stomach and bowels; and similar sounds in the heart and arteries. But the progress of chlorosis is generally slow; it occurs almost exclusively in women at the period of puberty, and often takes its rise without known cause. Anæmia, or simple deficiency of blood, generally commences rather suddenly, and is usually owing to spontaneous or secondary losses of blood; in short, in anæmia, we have simple diminution of the mass of the blood, while in chlorosis there is also a change in the chemical composition of that fluid.

China is the principal homœopathic remedy.

HYDRÆMIA,

Or, Watery Condition of the Blood.

This causes a peculiar kind of plethora or fulness of blood; although the patient is pale, languid, and dyspeptic, yet she has many of the symptoms which belong to plethora, such as dizziness, dazzling of the eyes, ringing in the ears, headache, difficulty of breathing, palpitations of the heart, throbbing of the arteries, flushing of the face, and drowsiness. The apparent superabundance of the blood is nothing more than an increase of the serous or watery parts of the blood, which fluid is actually impoverished and deprived of its nutritive qualities. Even BOERHAAVE regarded some cases of chlorosis as the result of an excess of serous blood; he says: the fluids are in excess over the solids, and their motion is retarded, because the mass to be moved is augmented, while the moving force is diminished; the body soon becomes inactive; the young girl becomes swelled and grows pale; for, to speak truly, she does not lose the red portion of her blood, but acquires more of the white than is necessary in proportion to the red.—BERNER, BUCHNER, and BEAN, have maintained the same view.

Arsenicum, Hellebore, Graphite, and Marsh Marigold, are the principal homœopathic remedies.

LEUCOCYTHEMIA,

Or, White Cell Blood.

The blood contains colored or red globules, and colorless globules, corpuscules, or cells. BENNETT has given the name Leucocythemia, or white cell blood, to a peculiar form of disorder, very much resembling anæmia and chlorosis, and in which these white or colorless globules exist in great excess in the blood. He thinks that the blood globules, especially the white ones, are formed in the lymphatic glands; in short, that the lymphatic glands secrete the blood corpuscules in the same manner as the testes secrete the semen and spermatazoa, the female breasts the globules of milk, or the salivary or gastric glands form the cells of the saliva or gastric juice. He repeats, that the blood corpuscles are originally formed in the lymphatic glandular system, and that the great majority of them, on joining the circulation, become colored by the addition of Iron, and by exposure to the oxygen in the lungs, and assumes that, in certain diseases and enlargements of the lymphatic glands, their cell elements are multiplied to an unusual extent, and find their way into the blood, causing a great increase in their white or colorless cells. *This is Leucocythemia.* The easiest way to detect the disease is, to obtain a drop of blood by pricking the finger of the patient with a needle, and then examining it under the microscope;

the yellow and colorless corpuscules are at first seen rolling confusedly together, and the excessive number of the latter is at once perceived; sometimes they are five times as numerous as in health.

This disease is very important, as it is rebellious to all allopathic treatment; BENNETT says, in no one instance has the condition of the blood been observed to undergo any marked improvement after the excess of white cells has been discovered in it.

Leucocythemia resembles chlorosis in some marked particulars:

1st. The fibrin is in excess, 7 times out of 9, varying from $\frac{3.2}{1000}$ to $\frac{9.08}{1000}$, while the natural standardard is only $\frac{3}{1000}$.

2. The serum or water is in excess, varying from $\frac{801}{1000}$ to $\frac{881}{1000}$, while the natural and healthy quantity is only $\frac{790}{1000}$.

3. The blood globules are diminished from the natural standard of $\frac{127}{1000}$ to $\frac{100}{1000}$, or even to $\frac{67}{1000}$, and in some few cases to $\frac{49}{1000}$.

The distinctive characters of the disease, are: enlargement of the spleen, and disease of the lymphatic glands; in 19 cases of leucocythemia, the spleen was found to be more or less enlarged in 16; in the same 19 cases, the lymphatic glands were more or less diseased in 11.

It is probable, however, that disease or disorder of the spleen also exists in chlorosis, and even that this may be the principal cause of the alteration in the blood; at least, ECKER and BECLARD have come to the conclusion that the blood globules are incessantly disintegrated or destroyed in the spleen. They base their opinion upon the following facts:

1st. The blood returned by the splenic vein, prior to its junction with the vena porta, contains a smaller proportion of blood globules than arterial blood, and even all kinds of venous blood; thus, the blood of the splenic vein contains only $\frac{128}{1000}$ of globules and fibrin, while that of the external jugular has as much as $\frac{141}{1000}$, the mammary artery $\frac{159}{1000}$, and the vena porta as much as $\frac{227}{1000}$. The deficiency of globules in the splenic vein can only be accounted for by the supposition that the blood globules are destroyed or disintegrated in the spleen.

2d. The quantity of albumen in the splenic vein is much greater than in any other blood-vessel; there are only $\frac{70}{1000}$ in the blood of the vena porta, $\frac{79}{1000}$ in that of the external jugular, $\frac{89}{1000}$ in that of the mammary artery, and as much as $\frac{124}{1000}$ in the blood of the splenic vein. BECLARD very justly concludes that the disappearance of the blood globules in the spleen can be conceived of with difficulty, without their principal element (albumen) being thus found to be present *in excess* in the splenic vein.

These facts render it very probable that excessive action of the spleen causes the diminution of the blood globules, and consequent pallor of the surface, in chlorosis, leucocythemia, and even in the paludal cachexia of fever and ague; all allied diseases. This supposition, that the spleen is involved in chlorosis, will account for the frequency, obstinacy, and severity of the chlorotic and hysterical pain in the left side, just under the left breast. Leucocythemia, then, would differ from chlorosis, principally in the additional disease of the lymphatic glands and system, which attend the former disease.

The principal homœopathic remedy against simple chlorosis is Plumbum; against leucocythemia, are, Natrum muriaticum, Iodine, Iodides of Iron and Lead, and Conium, or Belladonna.

Treatment.—TILT says, that chlorotic patients are notoriously fond of ease, and all they want is to be allowed to remain in a state of muscular quietude; but this desire must no more be listened to, than that of travellers yielding to the soporific effects of intense cold; for the habitually cold skin of chlorotic patients causes a half-poisoned state of the blood, by the retention of what should be excreted, and the imperfect oxygenation it undergoes; with this vitiated, and lympathic, and venous blood, the internal organs are overloaded [especially the spleen]. They should, therefore, be urged and enforced to exert themselves, so that the blood may circulate more rapidly, and thereby absorb that due quantity of oxygen which is necessary to impart to it those vital properties which excite all the organs to perform their proper functions. The limbs and body should be rubbed briskly once or twice a day, in order to solicit the blood to the surface; Dr. HOLLAND recommends the exercise of respiration, to invigorate the system and improve the blood, by a more perfect oxygenation of it, for, in chlorosis, the chest in general is scarcely seen to rise, and breathing must be very imperfectly performed. The use of an inhaling-tube is entirely unnecessary; the patient need only take long, and full, and deep breaths for several minutes, or 10 minutes in succession, several times a day. Reading aloud and singing are excellent exercises for the lungs.

PLUMBUM.

This is undoubtedly the most homœopathic remedy for chlorosis. To Dr. F. C. WINTER, of LUNENBURG, is due the credit of introducing this remedy into homœopathic practice. ANDRAL says, that the prolonged use of lead induces the same conditions of the blood as those we see in chlorosis; an interesting case, reported by TANQUEREL, shows how deceptively the disease produced by lead simulates chlorosis: A man, aged 21, of strong constitution, came under treatment for chlorosis, and great palpitation of the heart, following exposure to lead for 18 months. WINTER used it with success in cases of chlorosis marked by difficulty of breathing, constipation, dropsy of the feet, and unusual debility, in which the ordinary means, both homœopathic and allopathic had been tried without benefit; the obstinate, and almost invincible constipation, led him to use Plumbum, which proved of great service, not only in this, but against almost all the other concomitants of chlorosis. DRYSDALE has also used it, with marked benefit, in cases of chlorosis, after the more active state of disorder of the digestive organs has been subdued by other medicines, and the chief, or only symptoms which remain are: difficulty of breathing, obstinate constipation, muscular debility, and scanty or suppressed Menstruation.

According to WINTER, Plumbum is homœopathic when the

patient has a peculiar, pale, often waxy, greenish-yellow complexion, with a yellowish tinge of the whites of the eyes; when the eyes are deeply sunken and surrounded by dark, or blue circles; when the pulse is frequent, small, and soft; the patient being very dispirited, anxious, and despairing; also very feeble, with bewildering confusion and pain in the head; when the lips, gums, and inside of the mouth, are very pale, or bluish-gray, in color; when there is a want of appetite, or desire only for particular things; thirst, with burning in the stomach; eructations, nausea, vomiting, aching in the stomach, cramps in the bowels, obstinate constipation, alternating with diarrhœa; diminished secretion of urine; laborious or sighing respiration, with more or less oppression and tightness of the chest, with anxiety and palpitation of the heart; pains in the back, loins, and limbs, with great weariness and languor; coldness of the body, dropsy of the feet, and frequently a general and uniform dropsical swelling of the whole body.

It has also proved useful when there are intense headaches, noises in the ears, suppressed, scanty, or irregular Menstruation, with insurmountable indolence, great drowsiness, frequent yawning, great debility, softness and flaccidity of the muscles, and trembling of the limbs, sadness, love of solitude, absence of mind, and melancholy, the patient being shy, depressed, and indifferent to all things.

WINTER used it, with surprisingly good effects, in 7 cases.

NATRUM MURIATICUM.

According to PIORRY, this remedy, given in doses of from 4 to 8 drachms, effects very rapidly what no other succedaneum of Quinine, that he has tried, ever does, viz., a diminution of the size of the spleen. PIORRY promptly cured 6 out of 8 cases in which he tried it. Bathing with salt and water over the region of the spleen, or wearing a salt-bag there, or the use of warm or cold salt water baths, may also be useful. It may also prove useful in scrofulous cases, and in true leucocythemia. (See DUNSFORD's 15 cases of scrofula, cured by a trituration of sea salt: Brit. Jour. of Hom., vol. 3, p. 37.)

PULSATILLA

Is the most homœopathic remedy when the blood becomes deprived of many of its red globules, not by disease of the spleen or lymphatic glands, but by simple or scrofulous irritation of the mucous membranes and follicles of the stomach, bowels, air-tubes, or of other organs.

It has been recommended in many disorders of females, when attended with chills, or a persistent coldness, especially of the limbs, even when the temperature of the atmosphere is warm; under these circumstances, it will prove useful in chlorosis, menstrual colics, and in cramps of the stomach and bowels.

FLEISCHMANN gave it with success to a girl, aged 17, who had not yet menstruated, but was feeble, with a pale and puffed countenance; complained of fatigue of the whole body, especially of the legs and feet; whose appetite was diminished, tongue furred, taste in the mouth bad, with frequent eructations; breathing short and oppressed, especially after exercise, with strong pulsations of the heart, and distinct *bruit de diable* in the carotid arteries, the pulse being feeble and slow. She improved after 14 days' use of Pulsatilla, 4th decimal dilution, and seemed well in a month.

GUERARD gave it to a girl, aged 14, not yet menstruated, who was slightly chlorotic, had emaciated, was troubled with colics and constipation, nausea, loss of appetite, coated tongue, slight fever every evening, and with cramps in the feet and legs. *Pulsat* 30 was followed by an erysipelatous eruption upon the legs, and by Menstruation at the end of fifteen days, when she soon recovered her natural color and health. Pulsatilla 18 was also given by Dr. GUERARD, to a chlorotic young lady, aged 24, who was pale, sallow, and languishing, with uncertain and irregular Menstruation, troublesome bloating of the stomach and bowels, burning in those parts, and in the throat, vomiting after each meal, preceded by acrid risings. Bellad.

30, allayed the vomitings, and Pulsat. 18 then removed the rest of the complaint, so that she recovered her healthy color and strength, became free from acidity, and her digestion was good.

HENDERSON treated a lady, aged 27, of pretty full habit, with sallow complexion, whose menses had first been scanty and irregular for 6 months, then totally suppressed for 3 months, but finally had appeared scantily about a month before; she had taken Iron for 5 months without improvement, was rarely free from headache for more than a day or two, was very feeble, especially on attempting to walk, subject to difficulty of breathing and palpitation from the most ordinary exertion, and even while at rest; her lips were very pallid. She then spent 9 months in the country without medical treatment, and improved but little in health; the menses appeared only for 1 day at a time, at long intervals, and very scantily; she was last unwell about 9 weeks ago, scantily for the whole of 1 day, and a part of 2 others; her difficulty of breathing and palpitation were worse; the headaches recurred every 2 or 3 days; she slept badly, had very little appetite; her feet swelled at night; there was evident pulsation of the carotids, and a strong continuous chlorotic murmur in the right side of the neck; bowels regular.

Treatment.—Pulsatilla 12, twice a day; in 4 days she became unwell, and continued so for 3 days, with more discharge than she had had for 2 years, with some improvement to her general health. At the end of a month, *China* 12, and *Graphite* 30, morning and evening, were given, followed in 1 day by Menstruation more profuse than for years, and her headache left her, strength and appetite improved; but her breathing and color remained as before. *Ferrum* 18, and *Graphite* 20, morning and evening, at the end of 2 weeks more, when she still continued free from headache and was able to employ herself actively within doors. Then, Pulsatilla 6 was given, twice a day, with still greater improvement, so that she menstruated 4 entire days, with abundant secretion, and dyspnœa and palpitations finally lessened. Fifteen days after she commenced the use of Graphite 12, twice a day, for 20 days, when Pulsat. 6, twice a day, completed the cure. She was under treatment 5 months in all.

Dose.—See pages 64 and 95.

FERRUM.

This is the most decided and useful antipathic remedy, yet KNORRE says, that he has used it successfully in chlorosis, with vertigo, painful aching in the head and stomach, loss of appetite, sluggish bowels, paleness of the face and whole of the body, also of the lips and tongue; the menses being very scanty and resembling serum; emaciation, excessive weakness, especially of the knees; swelling and bloating of the face, hands, and especially of the feet; frequent chills and constant coldness; weak pulse.

The allopathic experience with the use of Iron is abundant and conclusive; most physicians agree in stating that a cure of chlorosis may generally be effected with it, in from 2 to 6 weeks; it has a peculiar power of increasing the richness and redness of the blood, and produces the effects which are most wanted in this disease, viz., an augmentation of the proportion of red corpuscules, and a diminution of the quantity of fibrine. The use of some preparation of Iron is the more required, as there is a positive deficiency of Iron in the blood in chlorosis. Thus, BECQUEREL and RODIER, in 1000 grammes of calcined healthy blood, found ½ a gramme of *Iron*; this 1000 grammes of healthy blood contained 141 grammes of blood globules. On the other hand, the proportionate quantity of Iron in 31 cases of chlorosis was also ⅓ of a gramme; but then there were only 91 grammes to the 1000 of blood globules, whence it has been assumed that the deficiency of red globules stands in a close relation and proportion to the diminished quantity of Iron in chlorosis.

In scrofulous cases and in chlorotic *Hyperhydræmia*, when there is considerable fulness of the system and a diminished proportion of blood globules, from retention in the blood of its watery parts, owing more to a deficient excretion from the skin and kidneys, than to an absolute diminution of the globules, the

Iodide of Iron has been found serviceable, as it seems to promote the secretions more than any other preparation of Iron, and sometimes acts as a diuretic. It is also useful when there are enlargements of the glands and tonsils; and is said to have brought on Menstruation when other preparations of Iron have been used for a considerable time without effect. WILLIAMS, from many comparative trials, thinks the Iodide the most speedily useful preparation; he has cured chlorosis with it in 3 weeks, and replaced extreme pallor with the rosy hue of health.

The young practitioner may easily be deceived in reading the glowing accounts of allopathic physicians, of the effects of Iron in chlorosis, into the belief that it is only requisite to give Iron in these cases, in order to effect a prompt and certain cure. But PETREQUIN has observed many cases of chlorosis, which have resisted Iron as obstinately as does the anæmia connected with cancer, or organic disease; other cases, again, after deriving a certain amount of benefit from Iron, remain stationary; and others again appear cured by it, but the cure is not permanent. The remedy required in these cases, according to PETREQUIN, is *Manganese;* he has proved that Manganese is a normal constituent of animal and vegetable tissues, and believes that, wherever Iron exists in appreciable quantity, Manganese co-exists with it. Hence he infers that Iron alone will not succeed in some blood-diseases, but requires the aid of Manganese.

Dose.—See page 57.

CARBON.

It is unnecessary to enter into a dull detail of the great homœopathicity of the carbonaceous remedies, viz., Sepia, Graphite, Carbo animalis, and Carb. vegetabilis, to chlorosis. In homœopathic practice, the remedies which act upon the carbon of the body, and the venous system are most relied upon in chlorosis; in allopathic practice, those remedies which act upon the oxygen and the arterial system are the favorites. In proof, however, of the homœopathicity of the carbonaceous remedies, we add the following: chlorotic anæmia affected universally the workmen in a coal-pit near Valenciennes, but only those who worked in a particular gallery or pit; all who had ever been in it suffered, although, perhaps not for 3 or 4 months after the exposure; the gallery was strongly impregnated with sulphuretted hydrogen, and *carbonic acid.* They had symptoms resembling those of menstrual colic in females, and abdominal congestion; viz: severe colics, tightness of the chest, palpitations, debility, and prostration; the colic pains lasted for 10 or 12 days, then the skin became blanched and sallow, the pulse quick and feeble; profuse sweats and great weakness finally set in. The illness often lasted for several months, and even for a year; and the colics sometimes returned frequently.

SABINA

Is the specific homœopathic remedy against menorrhagic-chlorosis, although Dr. WATZKE has used it successfully against chlorosis with amenorrhœa.

CASE 1. A girl, of strong constitution, aged 17, had had suppressed Menstruation and chlorosis, for 6 months; she suffered with violent giddiness, especially in the morning, and from exertion, so that she sometimes fell down; pressing pain in the forehead, singing in the ears, greenish-yellow acrid leucorrhœa, shortness of breath, palpitations of the heart, great tendency to perspire, heaviness and painful weariness of the limbs; her skin was pale, and appearance leucophlegmatic; she had a great desire for sour things, and for burnt coffee.

Treatment.—Pulsatilla was given for 3 weeks without benefit, then 1 drop Ol. Sabina in a drachm of sugar, was given in 1 or 2 grain doses, with rapid relief.

CASE 2. A girl, aged 16, not yet menstruated, had suffered for 3 years with headache; cachectic appearance, with dark circles around the eyes, toothache, tendency to nausea and vomiting, heartburn, dragging and griping pains in the abdomen, pressure downwards upon the genitaliæ, shortness of breath, palpitations, oppressive pain in the chest, weight in the legs, with pain in the thighs when walking, dragging and tearing pains in the limbs, particularly at night, debility, great drowsiness, and laziness.

Treatment.—Puls., Sepia, Kali, Ferrum, and Silex were given for 2 months without benefit; she then recovered under the use of Sabina, as directed for Case 1.

Dose.—See page 70.

CHINA

Is also homœopathic to anæmia and chlorosis from excessive lactation and Menstruation, although WATZKE gave it with success in

CASE 1. An unmarried lady, aged 30, of strong constitution and phlegmatic temperament, had complained for several months with oppression and heaviness of the head, loss of appetite, tightness and distension of the belly, pain in the sides, short and difficult breathing, pressure upon the chest, frequent palpitations, swelling of the legs up to the knees, great weakness, so that she could only walk with great difficulty; the menses were scanty and pale; she had some leucorrhœa; the patient, who had previously always been in good health, with a blooming complexion, had become pallid and bloated, and she, who had formerly been sprightly and good-humored, had become very cross and lachrymose.

Treatment.—The alternate use of Ferrum and Helleb. nig., 1st dilution, followed by China, 3d dilut., permanently restored the patient in 9 or 10 weeks.

CASE 2. Miss A., aged 21, of delicate frame, menstruated at 16, accompanied with intolerable headaches, for which she was repeatedly and profusely leeched; finally, all the signs of confirmed chlorosis set in.

Treatment.—Ferr., Puls., Coccul., Hep., Ignat., and Nux were given without benefit, for 2 months; then she was cured in 2 months by China 3, and she remained well for at least 3 years afterwards.

Dose.—See page 45.

DIFFICULT AND PAINFUL MENSTRUATION.

DYSMENORRHŒA.

In 300 cases of uterine disease, BENNETT met with 123 instances of painful Menstruation. MADDEN, in 180 cases, with 34; ASHWELL, in 810 cases, found only 10 with dysmenorrhœa, 19 with irritable uterus, and 74 with hysteria.

Several varieties of the disease are described by authors, viz.:

1. From stricture or narrowness of the canal of the neck of the womb.
2. Spasmodic stricture of the sphincter at the os internum, which is formed by a strong band of the circular muscular fibres of the cervix, and destined to close the uterus during the latter stages of pregnancy.
3. From croupous or dysenteric inflammation of the internal surface of the womb, leading to the formation of false membranes, which are expelled with great pain and difficulty.
4. From simple or rheumatic inflammation of the womb, especially of its neck.
5. From a nervous and spasmodic action of the muscular fibres of the womb. And,
6. From congestion of the womb.

Of BENNETT's 123 cases of painful Menstruation, 2 commenced at 10 years of age; 8 at 11 years; 17 at 12 years; also, 17 cases at 13 years; 22 at 14 years; 20 cases at 15 years; *only* 9 cases at 16; 11 at 17 years; 8 at 18 years; 5 at 19; and 1 at 20. Hence it would seem as if painful Menstruation is more frequently connected with an early appearance of the menses, than with a delayed. COLOMBAT even asserts, that the subjects of dysmenorrhœa are generally of a nervous or bilious temperament, of ardent feelings, and greatly addicted to coitus, although constitutions precisely the opposite of these are not exempt from it; and during an attack of the disease, they generally feel a sensation of heat in the neck of the womb, a kind of pruritus of the vagina, and spasmodic constriction of the vulva. It is but right to add that COLOMBAT often seems to take a blackguardly pleasure in making similar assertions, which are generally unfounded.

1. *Dysmenorrhœa from Stricture, or Narrowness of the Canal of the Neck of the Womb.*

Dr. MACKINTOSH was the first to draw attention to this form of the disorder; as early as 1823, after having frequently met with much difficulty and embarrassment in the treatment of some cases of dysmenorrhœa, he thought that he perceived the signs of stricture of the canal of the neck of the womb, and imagined that dilating it with the bougie might prove a method of relieving the pain of the patient. In the course of a few years, from 1826 to 1832, he met with 20 cases of dysmenorrhœa, which he treated in this way, 18 of them with the most marked success, and only 2 without benefit; 10 of the 18 were barren married women, of whom, 7 afterwards became with child; 8 were unmarried, or widows.

In some of these cases, the stricture is very great, the aperture of the mouth of the womb being so small as scarcely to admit a hog's bristle, others being just large enough for the introduction of a small silver probe. Dr. MEIGS cannot boast of success equal to that of MACKINTOSH, but the treatment has certainly been productive of advantage in several instances, especially in the persons of 2 married ladies, who were not only relieved of their painful Menstruation, but, though they never before had been pregnant, soon became with child.

RIGBY has, however, given the best description of obstructive dysmenorrhœa. He says, that the chief feature of this species of the disorder is, that the pain precedes the discharge; it varies in different individuals, sometimes coming on but a few hours before Menstruation; at other times, the patient may begin to suffer for days or even a week before the menstrual flow commences. These differences probably depend on the slowness or rapidity with which the secretion comes on, and somewhat upon the amount of irritability which the womb manifests on becoming distended with the menstrual fluid. Hence, when the secretion flows fast, and the uterus resents the accumulation within its cavity, there will probably be a sharp, but short attack of pain, for the rapid distension of the uterus, and its contractions, will cause severe suffering, while they will quickly produce the requisite amount of dilatation which will allow the fluid to pass out of the womb, and thus relieve the pain. In mild cases, a moderate amount of distension is sufficient to effect the necessary degree of dilatation of the mouth of the womb, and the accumulated fluid is discharged, with complete relief to the patient; but where the obstruction is greater, and produces greater resistance, the accumulation goes on, the pain becomes more severe, and then, as the womb is roused to contract upon the retained fluid, the patient will experience exacerbations of intense suffering, similar to the severe pain which is often seen in bad cases of abortion and early miscarriage, until after a long and agonizing struggle, the obstruction is surmounted, and the discharge takes place.—RIGBY.

In cases of obstructive dysmenorrhœa of this severe character, the uterine system, as well as the general health, is apt to suffer considerably; the womb becomes enlarged by this periodical distension, so that the ordinary internal measurement of its cavity may increase from 2½ inches to 3, or even more; and this enlarged cavity will often not clear itself entirely of the menstrual fluid, more or less of which is apt to be retained; after a time, the thinner portions are absorbed, leaving what remains, of a dark, thick, molasses, or tar-like consistence, which may only be evacuated at the next monthly period. Hence it is, that in passing the sound, or dilating the neck of the womb, a quantity of dark, brown, and slimy fluid frequently besmears the instrument, and the patient has a discharge of a similar character for a day or two afterwards, with much relief. The stomach, liver, and bowels are apt to become deranged, with more or less hæmorrhoidal congestion and loaded urine, and the tongue soon displays that dry, rough, short-napped, brownish fur, which so invariably attends uterine irritation.—RIGBY.

Obstructive dysmenorrhœa seldom continues for any length of time, without producing more or less ovarian irritation. The ovaries are well known to present a considerable degree of irritation and congestion at these times, even in a state of health; but, under such circumstances as those above mentioned, the congestion assumes more the character of inflammation, with great aggravation of the patient's sufferings There is severe pain in the groin, above Poupart's ligament, darting down the thigh; the part is very tender on pressure, and frequently feels to the patient as if swelled; finally, chronic inflammation of the ovary may be set up, and then is not unfrequently attended with severe menorrhagia.

RIGBY also says, that there is no doubt, that a large number of cases of obstructive dysmenorrhœa are due to an originally contracted state of the mouth of the womb, or of the canal of the neck of the womb, and accordingly we find, that in many or most of these cases, the patient has suffered at her menstrual periods, from their first commencement. In some cases, the pain and difficulty do not come on until some years after the first establishment of Menstruation, and in others, not until after marriage; in these cases, the principal part of the pain is owing to a congested or swollen state of the lining membrane, obstructing still farther an orifice or canal, which, though originally contracted, had nevertheless at one time allowed the discharge of the menstrual fluid without any peculiar difficulty. RIGBY also thinks that there can be but little doubt that dysmenorrhœa, in females with rheumatic-gouty constitutions, arises from a similarly congested, swollen, and irritated state of the mucous membrane lining the mouth and canal of the neck of the womb.

BENNETT says, that extreme dysmenorrhœa, from *congenital* contraction of the neck of the womb, is of rare occurrence, but admits that dilatation is sometimes the only means we have of remedying an extreme amount of suffering at the menstrual period. He gives the case of a young female, aged 22, who had suffered in the most excruciating manner at every menstrual period since the menses first appeared at the age of 18; the pain always continued without intermission, throughout the 3 days and nights that Menstruation lasted, and was of so severe a character, that she never closed her eyes, and was confined to bed the whole time. She had been almost constantly under medical treatment, without the least relief from antispasmodics, anodynes, or sedatives; even large doses of Opium were given without the slightest benefit.

Mechanical Treatment.—Dilatation was effected to a considerable extent in the course of 3 weeks, preceding the next menstrual period, by means of small sponge tents; the very next Menstruation was more abundant than usual, and she was entirely free from pain; the next period was also free from pain and she remained well. MEIGS prefers the use of a flexible block-tin bougie; if the instrument be somewhat curved, its apex will enter without difficulty, and should be passed slowly upwards to the distance of 1½ to 2 inches, and allowed to remain for a minute or two, and then withdrawn, to be followed by one of a larger size. If the instrument be too large, the patient will complain of a sense of aching in the womb; it is undesirable to cause any pain. This mode of treatment is evidently proper in some cases; the cause of the pain is evident and should be removed, for the cavity of a non-pregnant healthy womb will not contain more than 10 or 12 drops of fluid, and as soon as the menstrual secretion commences from the lining membrane of the womb, unless the blood finds free exit, it will distend the the uterus and give rise to great pain; as soon as the obstruction is overcome, the blood will escape freely and the pain ceases. RIGBY prefers the use of a peculiar dilator, the blades being made of well-tempered steel, and opened after being introduced into the canal of the cervix, and allowed to remain so for about a minute, thus rapidly effecting a considerable degree of dilatation, often with very striking relief, even when used but a short time before a menstrual period, the discharge appearing freely, with but little pain.

2. *From Congestion.*

BENNETT says, in those females in whom the womb is naturally predisposed to congestion, and in whom Menstruation is very abundant, and often preceded and followed by a white leucorrhœal discharge, Menstruation is apt to be painful, either for the first day, or throughout the entire period. In such women, the dysmenorrhœa is evidently functional, and the result of the distension caused by the excessive congestion, combined perhaps with a peculiar susceptibility of the uterine nerves.

WHITEHEAD has paid most attention to congestive dysmenorrhœa; he says, it consists essentially in a state of vascular hypertrophy of the womb and its appendages, and is associated, to a greater or less extent, with a similar condition of the portal circulation generally. The whole, or a considerable portion of the womb is found to be large and weighty, attended with some prolapsus; the neck of the womb is tumid, occasionally excoriated, or presenting a granular surface, and generally less firm than natural; some retroversion or anteversion is apt to be present, causing frequent desire to empty the bladder, or pain and difficulty in evacuating the bowels, while it increases the pain of Menstruation by narrowing the canal of the neck of the womb, owing to the bent state of the part in this displacement. The walls of the vagina are apt to be relaxed, and the vulva may be swollen and marked with venous distension; the upper part of the thighs may also be marked by enlarged veins, and piles may be present. This form is more frequent in the married than in the virgin state, and it often exists in the barren, and in those who have experienced frequent abortions.

Bellad., Stramon., Sabina, and Borax are the principal remedies.

3. *From Spasmodic Contraction.*

This may arise from a spasmodic contraction of the whole of the womb, or merely of that kind of muscular sphincter, which exists at the os internum, formed by a strong band of the circular muscular fibres of the neck of the womb. In some cases, this may merely be a nervous or muscular affection, but very frequently the spasm is caused by congestive, inflammatory, or rheumatic irritation of these parts.

Nux, Ignatia and Secale are the principal homœopathic remedies.

4. *From Inflammation and Ulceration of the Neck of the Womb.*

Bennett is, of course, the enthusiastic advocate for the frequency of this form of the disorder. He says it generally exists when Menstruation which was originally easy, or but slightly painful, finally becomes extremely so; such a change does not take place without a cause, and that cause is, generally speaking, inflammation and ulceration of the neck of the womb; dysmenorrhœa being one of the most prominent and most ordinary symptoms of that disease. This remark, he insists, applies to to the virgin as well as to the married female, and is of extreme importance, as affording a key to those extreme cases of dysmenorrhœa, accompanied by spinal irritation and hysterical convulsions, which appear to resist every form of allopathic treatment, and are alike distressing to the patient, her friends, and medical attendant. Since he has ascertained this fact, nearly all the cases of *extreme* dysmenorrhœa in the unmarried female, that have come under his notice, have proved to be of this description, and, however impracticable before, have yielded as soon as proper treatment has been adopted. These cases, he says, are easily distinguished from those caused by contraction of the neck of the womb; for in the latter, the patient is free from pain, except at the menstrual period, but when there is inflammation and ulceration, there is not the same immunity from pain during the interval.

The principal homœopathic remedies are Arsenicum, Aurum muriaticum, Borax, used both locally and internally, and the Chloride of Platina.

5. *From Ovarian Irritation.*

LOOMIS adopts TILT's ovarian theory of many uterine diseases, and of dysmenorrhœa among the rest, with considerable enthusiasm. The subject is now so hackneyed, that I merely refer to it here, in order to point out the most homœopathic remedies, when the ovaries are decidedly involved.

Argentum nitricum is indicated when the menses are profuse and painful, with pains especially in the small of the back, groin, and ovaries.

Granatum, when Menstruation lasts but a short time, is profuse, with colic, and pressing pains in the small of the back, groins and ovaries.

Borax, when the menses are attended with spasmodic and lancinating pains in the groins and ovaries.

Kali hydriodicum, when there are aching pains in both groins and ovaries, and small of the back.

Cantharides, Graphite, and Staphysagria also deserve attention, when the ovaries are disordered.

6. *Pseudo-membranous Variety.*

This has generally been regarded as owing to a peculiar or croupous inflammation of the lining membrane of the womb; but POUCHET states, that in all females, even in virgins, a delicate decidual membrane or cast is formed in the cavity of the womb at every Menstruation, and is thrown off about the 10th day. If this be so, the deciduous pseudo-membranes of dysmenorrhœa may be considered as merely an exaggeration of a natural condition, which, however, may be still further increased by the superaddition of croupous inflammation. BENNETT, of course, believes, or rather assumes, that the formation of these membranes coincides almost invariably with the present or past existence of uterine inflammation; he, doubtless, can see further into a mill-stone, or the womb, than anybody else, but that does not prevent him from being as absolutely ignorant of the appearances of inflammation as was BROUSSAIS. Still, he has grace enough to admit that the removal of the inflammatory disease does not always free the patient from the liability to the formation of pseudo-membranous casts.

The presence of these false membranes aggravates the patient's distress considerably; their expulsion is always preceded by an increase of the uterine pains, and not unfrequently by tormina similar to labor-pains, which are evidently occasioned by the violent efforts of the womb to get rid of the membranes and casts formed in its cavity; that the difficulty of expulsion is partly the cause of the severe contractions and pains, is proved by the fact that they have repeatedly been relieved by dilating the canal of the mouth of the womb during the interval of Menstruation, and this in females who still continued to expel false membranes, even after all visible disease of the womb had disappeared.

Treatment.—It is evident that mechanical and general treatment will not remove this peculiar disorder; as we know of no homœopathic remedies for pseudo-membranous irritation, or croupous inflammation of the uterus in particular, it may be allowable to use the true croup remedies; thus, we will at least use remedies which are homœopathic to the nature of the disease, even if they have no specific relation to the locality. Bromine, Bichromate of Potash, Ammonium causticum, and Cantharides may be used with much prospect of success, especially as the latter also act specifically upon the uterine organs.

In the cases reported by Beauvais, Pulsatilla alone cured 3 cases; Puls. and Nux, 1 case; Puls. and Cocc., 1 case; Puls. and Sulph., also 1 case; Cocculus alone, 2 cases; Coccul. and Puls., 1 case; Graphite and Lycopod., 1 case; Graph. and Baryt. c., 1 case; Nux was used in 3 cases; Veratrum, Secale, Calcarea, Lachesis, Ignat., Conium, Platina, and Crocus, each in 1 case; Sulphur in 2 cases.

ACONITE.

Loomis recommends this remedy when the dysmenorrhœa arises from an inflammatory condition of the womb or ovaries, with violent fever, dry and burning heat of skin, excessive thirst for cold drinks, redness and heat of the face; distension of the abdomen, with tenderness to touch. It may also be suitable in alternation with Colchium, Bryonia, or Guaiacum, where painful Menstruation arises from a rheumatic affection of the womb.

Dose.—See page 36.

AMMONIUM CARBONICUM

Is also recommended by LOOMIS as most adapted to the inflammatory variety; the Ammonium causticum, we have already seen, is homœopathic to the pseudo-membranous form. It is said to be most indicated when painful Menstruation is attended with swelling, itching, and burning of the sexual organs, or excoriation of these parts, especially when the menses occur too soon, and are too copious, dark in color, and acrid; or if there be pain in the loins and colic, with pressing-down pain, &c. COLOMBAT recommends the Acetate of Ammonia; he says that it produces a rapid sedative action upon the womb, and relieves the painful tormina which attends the discharge; but if too much of it be given, it is apt to cause scanty Menstruation.

Dose.—Same as for Iodine and Phosphor. (See page 81.)

BELLADONNA

Is said by LOOMIS to be indicated in the inflammatory variety, although it may prove useful in some cases of the neuralgic form; it is, however, best suited to the congestive and spasmodic varieties. In fact, he proceeds to recommend it, when there is congestive enlargement of the womb, or falling of that organ, with menstrual colic and spasms, with labor-like pains. It is not generally known, that the so-called bearing-down pains are often merely a tenesmus of the os and cervix uteri; it is in these cases that Bellad. is so useful. HOLMES, of Mississippi, thinks that *Bellad.*, if rightly used, never fails to relieve the pain of dysmenorrhœa, and render Menstruation regular, free, and healthy; he thinks that it acts specifically upon the womb, relieves its pains and spasms, increases the flow, dilates the canal of the neck, and thus permits coagulæ and membranes to pass without the least inconvenience to the patient; but he uses $\frac{1}{3}$ grain doses of the extract.

Dose.—See page 40.

BRYONIA

Is a valuable adjunct in the rheumatic variety, especially if the symptoms of rheumatism of the womb be well marked, in addition to rheumatic pains about the head or chest, with short, dry cough, and frequent bleeding from the nose, or rheumatic pains and swellings of one or more joints or limbs.

Dose.—See page 41.

CALCAREA

Is recommended when the breasts are apt to be swollen and painful during Menstruation, with headache, colic, cramp-like pains in the region of the kidneys, acidity of the stomach, high-colored and acid urine, with chronic inflammation and swelling of the womb.

Dose.—See page 48.

BORAX

Has long been used in Germany to produce uterine contractions, and to facilitate the excretion of the lochia and menstrual fluid; it is the principal remedy against that aphthous and granular affection of the mouth and neck of the womb, which has led to so much abuse of the speculum and digital examination by Bennett and others. Bennett has lately found out that it is homœopathic and curative to membranous dysmenorrhœa. He gives the case of a woman, aged 26, subject for two years, since marriage, to painful Menstruation; the menses were regular as to time, but usually lasted a week, and were attended with such great suffering that she had always been compelled to lie down for the greater part of that time; the discharges were generally very dark in color, and mixed with clots of blood and numerous flakes of whitish membrane; in the intervals, there was more or less leucorrhœa, with dull aching pain in the lower part of the back; her tongue was redder than natural; pulse 96, and sharp. She had never conceived, and had been subjected to a great variety of treatment, with very little advantage. After taking the Biborate of Soda for 20 days, Menstruation occurred with very little pain, and was unmixed with either shreds or flakes; during the whole period she had been able to pursue her usual avocations, and had enjoyed a degree of comfort to which she had been a stranger for years; the next month she also menstruated without material suffering, the aching in her back had also disappeared, together with a chronic cough, which had persisted for several months.

It is thought to be especially adapted when there is slight fever, pain in the loins, and the expulsion of shreds and flakes of lymph.

Dose.—Same as for Calcarea. (See page 48.)

CROCUS,

Coffea, and Chamomilla, are admirable palliatives when frequent and profuse Menstruation is attended with great pain.

Dose.—See pages 43 and 55.

COCCULUS

Is generally regarded as the principal homœopathic remedy against menstrual spasms and colic; Loomis thinks it is more appropriate in the neuralgic than the inflammatory variety; but it, like Nux and Ignatia, is probably more homœopathic to the spasmodic form than any other. It is especially indicated when there is menstrual colic with cramps in the womb, early and profuse Menstruation with much pain, and followed by a sanious leucorrhœa during the interval. The indications for Nux and Ignatia are too well known to require repetition here.

Dose.—See page 57.

PHOSPHORUS

Is most homœopathic when there is excessive ovarian and sexual irritation, with inflammation of the ovaries and neck of the womb, the menses being profuse, and long continued, preceded by an acrid leucorrhœa, and accompanied with colic and cutting pains in the bowels, back-ache, and pains extending from the vagina up into the womb. Platina is recommended under nearly the same circumstances.

Dose.—See page 81.

PULSATILLA

Is used very frequently in dysmenorrhœa, especially when the menses are scanty or suppressed, the patient being rheumatic, or subject to a leucorrhœa of a corrosive and burning nature, and thick like cream.

Dose.—See page 93.

SECALE

Is decidedly the most homœopathic remedy in spasmodic dysmenorrhœa; it has been very rarely used, however, especially by those who pride themselves much more upon giving infinitessimal doses of some inert remedy, than upon always giving the most homœopathic remedy.

Dose.—See page 104.

SEPIA AND SULPHUR

Have been used in dyscratic and rheumatic cases.

Dose.—See pages 97 and 98.

UNNATURAL OR DEPRAVED MENSTRUATION.

I apply this rather rude name to that class of cases in which there is a decided alteration in the color, consistence, and odor of the menstrual secretion.

In 181 cases of uterine disease, MADDEN met with 19 instances in which the menses were too pale, and 8 in which they were too dark.

Dulcamara is said to be indicated when Menstruation is retarded, and the discharge is watery; *Ferrum acet.*, when menses are delayed, with a scanty discharge of watery blood; *Sulphur*, when the menstrual discharge is too pale; *Stramonium*, when it is watery; *Pulsatilla*, when pale and watery.

China is said to be homœopathic when there is a discharge of clots of black blood; *Ignatia*, when menses are black, scanty, and fetid; *Nux juglans*, when premature Menstruation is attended with pressing pain in the womb, and expulsion of blackish coagulæ; *Cantharides*, when menses are too profuse, early, and dark; *Pulsatilla*, when the blood is viscid, thick, clotted, and black; *Ignatia*, when lumps of coagulated blood are expelled; *Conium*, when the discharge is brownish in color; *Ammon. carb.*, when it is black.

Sulphur has been recommended when menses are profuse, with an acrid smell; *Bellad.*, in profuse Menstruation, when the blood smells badly; *Ignatia*, when menses are scanty, black, and fetid; *Sarsaparilla*, when they are scanty and acrid, so as to excoriate the inner side of the thighs: *Kreosote*, when menses occur too soon, with a discharge of acrid-smelling, bloody ichor; *Phosphor*, when the menstrual discharge has an offensive odor; *Sulphur*, when it is thick and acrid; *Rhus tox.*, when the menstrual blood is so acrid as to cause a severe smarting pain in the vulva; *Kali carb.*, when it is acrid and pungent, making the thighs sore; *Carb. veg.*, when it is acrid and corrosive.

LAST MENSTRUATION.

CHANGE OF LIFE.

The most common time for the cessation of the menses and change of life is between the 40th and 50th years; but, like the first appearance, so the cessation of Menstruation varies in different females, and is in subordination to the temperament, constitution, climate, and habit of life of the female; as a general rule, however, there is a certain relation between the periods of the first and last Menstruations, for the cessation occurs at a later period in proportion as the first appearance was less precocious.

BRIERE DE BOISMONT, in 183 cases, found two instances in which Menstruation ceased at 21 years of age; 1 case each at the 24th, 26th, 27th, 28th and 29th years of age; 3 cases at 31 years; 2 at 32 years; 4 at 34; 6 at 35; 7 at 36; 4 at 37; 7 at 38; 1 at 39; 18 at 40 years; 10 at 41; 7 at 42; 4 at 43; 13 at 44; 13 at 45; 9 at 46; 13 at 47; 8 at 48; 7 at 49; 12 at 50; 4 at 51; 8 at 52; 2 at 53; 5 at 54; 2 each at 55, 56 and 57 years; and 1 at the 60th year of age. Hence, of 183, in 7 it occurred between the 55th and 60th year of age; in 31 cases between the 50th and 55th years; in 50 cases between 45 and 50; in 52 cases between the 40th and 45th year; in 25 cases, from the 35th to 40th year; in 9 cases from the 30th to 35th year; in 7 cases from the 20th to the 30th year.

ROBERTON in 77 females, found 1 case to cease Menstruation at 35 years; 4 at 40 years; 1 each at 42 and 43; 3 at 44; 4 at 45; 3 at 47; 10 at 48; 7 at 49; 26 at 50; 2 at 51; 7 at 52; 2 each at 53 and 54; 1 at 57; 2 at 60; and 1 at 70 years of age.

ROBERTON also gives 13 instances of late Menstruation in Hindoo women, viz.: 2 cases still menstruated at 56 years of age; and 1 case each at 57, 58, 59, 60, 63, 64, 65, 67, 68, and 80 years of age.

In 2 Hindoo women, who commenced to menstruate at 11 years, menses ceased at 37 and 42. Of 6 women who commenced at 12 years, 2 ceased at 38, and 1 each at 40, 46, 49 and 52 years. Of 15 females who commenced at 13 years of age, 1 ceased at 40; 2 at 41; 1 each at 43, 45, 46 and 47; 4 at 48; 1 each at 50, 52 and 54. Of 18 cases which commenced at 14 years of age, 1 each ceased at 34 and 37, 40 and 41 years; 2 at 42; 1 at 43; 2 at 44; 1 at 47; 4 at 50; 1 each at 51, 54 and 58 years. Of 5 cases which commenced at 15 years, 1 ceased at 30; 1 at 40; 2 at 41; and 1 at 45. Of 2 cases which commenced at 16 years, 1 ceased at 45, the other at 46. Of 4 cases commencing at 17, 1 each ceased at 41, 43, 44 and 48 years. Of 2 cases commencing at 18, 1 ceased at 46, the other at 47.

BENNETT met with 2 females who commenced their menstrual life at 11 years, one of whom ceased menstruating at 47 years, the other between 40 and 50; 1 who began at 13 was still regular at 47; 1 at 14 ceased at 44; of 3 at 15, 1 each ceased at 48, 49 and 54 years; 1 at 16 ceased at 50; 5 at 18 ceased, 1 each at 41, 45 and 48, and 2 at 50 years; 2 at 19 years ceased, 1 at 44, the other at 50; of 2 at 20, 1 ceased at 50, the other at 53. On the other hand, BENNETT met with 1 case which commenced Menstruation at 11 years, and was still menstruating at 50; of 3 at 12 years, 1 each was still regular at 47 and 49, and the other at 56; of 7 beginning at 13 years, 3 were still menstruating at 47 years, and 1 each at 45, 50 and 52 years; of 2 commencing at 14, 1 was still regular at 45, and the other at 48; of 4 cases at 15, 2 were still regular at 47, and 1 each at 45 and 48; 1 case at 17 was still regular at 49; and 2 cases at 18 still menstruated at 46 and 51 years.

ROBERTON assumes that Menstruation always continues as late as the power of conception, and gives a table of 10,000 pregnant women, 436 of whom were over 40 years of age, viz.: 101 in their 41st year; 113 in their 42d; 70 in the 43d; 58 in the 44th; 43 in the 45th; 12 in the 46th; 13 in the 47th; 8 in the 48th; 6 in the 49th; 9 in the 50th; 1 each in their 52d, 53d, and 54th years. He also met with 3 women who had children at advanced ages, one in her 50th, another in the 51st, and the 3d in her 53d year; in all of whom Menstruation continued up to the period of conception. COLOMBAT mentions some curious cases of late pregnancy and Menstruation, viz., 1 case in which a woman was delivered in her 62d year; another in her 67th. HALLER mentions a woman still regular at 70, and brought to bed with child at that age. COLOMBAT saw a female who was very regular, and confined at 61 years of age; another who commenced Menstruation at 18, and continued regular up to the 73d year; while ORFILA gives the case of a woman who became pregnant with her first child at the age of 47, then had 7 children, the last when she was 60, remained regular until she was 99, and died at the age of 114.

Menstruation ceases abruptly in some women; gradually in others. TILT thinks that it terminates gradually in about 39 per cent.; by a succession of floodings in 19 per cent.; by a terminal flooding in 14 per cent.; by alternations of slight and considerable discharges in 10 per cent.; by a sudden stoppage in 18 per cent.

The gradual termination is the most frequent, and is, of course, attended with the least disturbance of health. A terminal flooding is often mistaken for miscarriage, and the sudden stoppage of the function deserves more attention than it has received, because it happens more frequently than is commonly supposed at an early period of life, and then is often mistaken for accidental suppression, and treated as such. Sudden cessation is also not unfrequently mistaken for pregnancy, especially if there is some amount of swelling of the abdomen and breasts, with secretion of milk, and other sympathetic disturbance, of which time only can show the fallacy.—TILT.

Sudden cessation often takes place thus: the person having arrived at the usual age, the expected Menstruation is prevented by cold, fright, or some illness; these accidents would have been followed, earlier in life, by a return of Menstruation after their removal; but it is not so now; nature seizes this opportunity to put and end to the function altogether, and many patients are thus dealt with, without experiencing any inconvenience. In *gradual* extinction, one period is missed, and then there is a return; a longer time elapses, and there is, perhaps, an excessive flow; afterwards, some months may pass away without any reappearance; then there may be a scanty secretion, followed perhaps by flooding; and finally the secretion becomes so scanty and so slightly bloody as scarcely to attract notice, and then disappears forever.—ASHWELL.

After a long period of cessation, the flow may reappear and return regularly for months and years, without, however, always indicating a return of procreative power. In some women, after cessation, the stock of vital productivity is fairly exhausted; but in most there is a superabundant nervous energy, or an excess of blood; for that supply, which was formerly sufficient for the maintenance of both mother and offspring, can now only be expended on the woman's frame.

Tilt also thinks that it is an important point to be remembered by women, that in proportion as their sufferings were protracted previous to the healthy establishment of Menstruation, so may they, in general, expect its cessation to be attended with a corresponding period and intensity of suffering. But it must not also be inferred, that those who have suffered little or none at its establishment, have no illness to expect, and therefore need take no precautions. Another fact, equally interesting and important to be known, is, that, in general, those diseases which precede the first appearance of Menstruation may possibly precede its cessation. Thus, Albert has observed some skin diseases to appear twice only in life, viz.: before the first appearance of Menstruation, and again at its cessation. Sir Henry Marsh noticed, that women, in whom the establishment of puberty had been preceded by repeated nose-bleedings, experienced the same accident as a prominent symptom of cessation. Tilt has several times seen both *first* and *last* Menstruation preceded in the same person by an abundant eruption of boils, frequently by continued diarrhœa, and still oftener by a great amount of pseudo-narcotism and hysteria.

Tilt also regards it as another indication useful to women, that, whenever irregular Menstruation is attended with a sinking feeling at the pit of the stomach, with flushes of heat and perspirations, even though their age may only be between 30 and 40, it is a warning of the commencement of the change of life. The usual concomitants of Menstruation are variously affected in different cases; in 64 cases out of 100, the patients generally had headache, sick headache, hysteria or pseudo-narcotism, at each menstrual period; and these symptoms were aggravated in 36 per cent. at the change of life; they remain unchanged in 18 per cent., were diminished in 10 per cent.

Tilt often refers to a train of symptoms, which he terms pseudo-narcotism; in the young girl, just before Menstruation, it consists of headache, dizziness, heaviness, dulness of intellect, tendency to sleep, &c. With a wonderful uniformity of language, changing girls will speak of a heaviness in the head, stupid feeling, stupid headache, feeling heavy for sleep; of being drowsy; of the possibility of sleeping anywhere, while at work, or standing; of feeling lost or bewildered; of losing their wits or memory for a time; of dimness of the eyes, or momentary loss of sight; of falling down while stooping; of involuntarily dropping any article which they may have in their hands; of forgetting, when sent on an errand, what they were sent for, and then being obliged to stand still and make an effort to recollect. Similar signs of pseudo-narcotism are apt to appear at the change of life; some women acquire an habitual giddiness, an uncertain and tottering gait, a vacancy of feature, a dull and drowsy expression of the eye. The more ordinary symptoms are: a great tendency to sleep, an uneasy sensation of weight in the head, a feeling as if a cloud or cobweb required to be brushed from the brain, disinclination for any exertion, and a diminution in the powers of memory, and of the mind. Some become exceedingly depressed and melancholic, sit in an indolent posture, look gloomy, hardly speak at all, and live under the impression that some evil is about to befall them; they are apt to be suspicious and undecided in all their movements.—Tilt.

The same author also places much stress upon the feelings of sinking or depression at the pit of the stomach, not an actual pain, but an irritating and tormenting sense of a want of support, or of emptiness; these feelings are associated with hot flushes, burning heats, and, in fact, are the harbingers of flushes and suffusions of the cheeks; on the subsidence of the heats, the skin breaks out into perspirations, either gentle or drenching, sometimes hot, at others cold and clammy.

Tilt met with these sensations of faintness, exhaustion, and sinking at the pit of the stomach, in 26 cases out of 100;

With heats and flushes in	38	"	"
" perspirations in	30	"	"
" sweats	16	"	"

These flushes and perspirations are the means by which nature relieves the system of the fluids, which used to be discharged every month; the heats, flushes, and gentle perspirations often prevent internal disease; in about 16 per cent., the sweats, by their amount, form a disease of themselves, without relieving the patient as well as a more moderate exhalation; these heats, flushes, and perspirations have been known to continue to appear several times a day for 10 or 16 years after the cessation of Menstruation. Tilt has known the perspirations to become so profuse that the drops accumulated as fast as they were wiped off the face, and the clothes were always wet; and when in bed the sufferer was afraid of turning, for fear that she should be chilled by the damp cold in the immediate vicinity of the body.

After cessation, it is not uncommon to have a continuance, or even an augmentation of the pains, by which Menstruation was usually attended, and the patients need not fancy from this circumstance alone that serious disease is impending. These pains are, in a large proportion of cases, merely nervous, and doubtless are meant to warn women that a certain degree of prudence is necessary while they last.

Pains in the back existed in	70	per cent.;
" " were increased in	46	"
" " remained the same in	17	"
" " were lessened in	7	"

Pains in the lower part of the body, of a bearing-down character, were present in 51 per cent.; which were increased in 30, remained unchanged in 10, and were lessened in 9.

Flooding occurred in 27 cases out of 100 about the time of the change of life; this symptom, which at other times would be considered pernicious, is not so alarming at this period, and need not be interfered with, unless it is too much for the patient's strength; but if these profuse flows occur too often, or are too abundant, and last very long, the woman should not allow her health to be completely ruined by this constant drain, but should apply for relief.

At the change of life, the blood, instead of being directed to the skin, as shown by the flushes and perspirations, or to the womb, as proved by the occurrence of floodings, or profuse leucorrhœa, may be turned towards the internal surface of the body, the stomach, liver, or bowels. BUTLER LANE says, it is very common to find severe biliary derangement at, or about the change of life; the patient is apt to have a bitter, oily taste in the mouth, a sensation of burning in the throat, frontal headache, nausea, and even vomiting, high-colored urine, bilious passages, furred tongue, and bilious tint of the skin. Diarrhœa is apt to come on, either irregularly, or quite regularly every month. Piles are also apt to come on, for the first time, about the change of life, or to be increased if they have already been present. Still, diarrhœa is much less frequent at the time of cessation, than as a symptom of regularly established Menstruation. TILT met with it in only 8 per cent. in the former case, while it occurred in 88 instances out of 161 regularly menstruating women; in those cases in which it was present, it preceded the menstrual flow in 45 cases, accompanied it in 31, both preceded and attended it in 10, and in 2 cases it followed the monthly flow for 2 days. As a general rule, however, when diarrhœa has habitually accompanied Menstruation, there is at the change of life a gradual diminution of both discharges, the cessation of one marking the termination of the other.

On the other hand, CORFE, of the Middlesex Hospital, thinks that there is no organ in the female economy which so readily partakes of disturbance from uterine irregularities, as the liver; and the instances are not few, where protracted bleeding from the womb at the change of life, which has resisted all other treatment, will yield to remedies directed to the liver. In such cases, the womb takes on a vicarious action for the liver; and so long as this organ is allowed to remain in its torpid condition, so long will the womb continue to pour out an undue quantity, or an altered quality, of dark, venous fluid, and the patient becomes enfeebled, harassed, and distressed; piles, also, are not unfrequently induced. But, oftentimes, no sooner do the remedies tell upon the hepatic branches of the portal system, than the uterine portion of the same system becomes relieved from its congested state, and the uterine discharge is quickly subdued. The alvine evacuations are usually offensive, fetid, and so dark, that CORFE has known them to partake of the character of the motions of a patient with malæna for several days together; and he is inclined to think that it is from the fact that physicians so rarely look at these excretions themselves, that many cases of this disorder are misunderstood, and therefore mismanaged. Whenever the urine ceases to deposit lithates, and becomes of a pale canary color, and the evacuations from the bowels present a healthy appearance, and cease to emit a penetrating fetor, then there will be a corresponding amelioration in the state of the patient; her spirits will become more buoyant, her mind less distressed, her appetite more equable, and her whole frame less heavy and weary.

Treatment.—ASHWELL says, that no more serious mistake can be made than to attribute any of the symptoms of this period to debility rather than to repletion, without the most accurate inquiry. Let it be remembered that an accustomed evacuation is about to cease, or has finally disappeared, and that hence the probability is that the system is oppressed, and that the weakness is apparent, rather than real. If, for instance, because there is languor and inactivity, a slow pulse, torpid bowels, and depression of mind, stimulants and generous diet be allowed, some important organ will be sure to suffer. A light and nutritious, but not a full diet, should be allowed, with little or no wine, and no malt liquors. Owing to the distressing sensations commonly felt at this time, small quantities of spirits are sometimes prescribed, and are always gladly taken by the patient; but their good effects are only temporary, while their permanent influence is most mischievous. Veal, pork, salt meat, fried and boiled fish, tea, pastry, and made dishes, or ragouts, wine, bottled beer, or any liquid containing free acid, or gaseous matter, seem to aggravate the disorder in a marked degree. Beef, mutton, roast or boiled, boiled fish, fresh game, or cocoa, form the best diet; and CORFE is quite enthusiastic about the benefits to be derived from taking half a dozen oysters, without any other food or additions, such as pepper, vinegar, &c., or even bread, upon an empty stomach, as for luncheon, for instance; their alkalescent character often removes the morbid acidity of the stomach, and restores its tone and vigor.

In accordance with these views, LEADAM recommends Aconite as the most soothing of all medicines at the climacteric period, especially if the patient be robust or plethoric, and if there be any evidence of local or general increased action. PULTE recommends Pulsatilla and Lachesis as the most important remedies.

When there is great nervous irritability, Aconite, Coffea, Ignatia, and Pulsatilla are recommended.

If there be congestion of the head or abdomen, with fulness, tension and pressure internally, attended with lumbar and sacral pains, LEADAM suggests the use of Belladona, to be followed in some cases by Hepar. sulph., and Sulphur. TILT has hit upon the use of *Sulphur* during the climacteric period; he says, that it owes its chief value, in diseases of cessation, not to its laxative properties, but to another action, much more difficult to understand, and which has long rendered it so valuable both in hæmorrhoidal affections, where there is an undue action of the intestinal capillaries, and in affections of the skin, marked by a morbid activity of the cutaneous capillaries. Whether Sulphur cures by acting on the nerves, or on the blood-vessels, or by modifying the composition of the blood itself, TILT finds it difficult to decide, but it certainly cures many of the affections of changing women. It forms part of many popular remedies for the infirmities of old age; it has been recommended by HUFELAND, and is lauded by Dr. Day, in his work "On the Diseases of Old Age"; but its utility is not generally known, except to the homœopathist, in many of the derangements of the menstrual function, at whatever period of life they may occur, and particularly at the change of life, where, if required, its action may be continued with impunity for months and years. It is particularly serviceable against bilious derangements, piles, sweats, and flushings.

If there be a burning sensation in the head, with bleeding from the nose, Crocus and Carb. veg. may be required.

If there has been menorrhagia from congestion of the womb, and great debility has ensued, the remedies for profuse Menstruation (see pages 36 to 73) should be used, among which, Aurum, *Aloe*, Chamomilla, China, Calcarea, *Crocus*, Ferrum, Kreosote, Platina, Sabina, Secale, and Sulphur, deserve most attention.

If nervous faintness and exhaustion are present, Valerian, Veratrum, Nitric acid, Kali carb., and Moschus are recommended by LEADAM.

Cocculus is also recommended as of use in the spasmodic attacks, seated either in the uterus or ovaries, especially when attended with bilious vomiting, or nausea.

Ruta is supposed to be particularly useful against the pains in the small of the back, sacrum, and os coccygis.

Nux, Pulsat., and Bryon. are the chief remedies against the dyspeptic symptoms.

Aloe is one of the best remedies against long continued flowing, and against bleeding piles. TILT says, he has never seen hæmorrhoidal affections caused by the frequent use of Aloes, but he has seen them relieved by it, and his experience is corroborated by that of GIACOMINI, AVICENNA, STAHL, and CULLEN. I have made frequent and successful use of Aloes and Iron, against profuse and long continued flowing, and against bleeding piles.

The profuse perspirations and flushings may be treated by Aconite, Opium, Sulphur, Arnica, &c.

Sudden suppression should be met by the remedies for the suppression of the menses, (see pages 112 to 116).

Arsenicum and China are the best remedies against chills and sweats.

Sabina and Bovista, against profuse leucorrhœa.

Sabina, Cuprum, and Phosphor., against the tendency to chronic bilious derangement.

INDEX.

K

Just Published, the Third Volume of JAHR'S NEW MANUAL; *or the largest*

REPERTORY OF THE HOMŒOPATHIC MATERIA MEDICA; By Dr Ch. Hempel. This is the most important and complete work ever published, and *indispensable* for every physician. 1853. Price $6.

LAURIE, Dr. J., HOMŒOPATHIC DOMESTIC MEDICINE, with the Treatment and Diseases of Females, Infants, Children and Adults. 7th American dition, much enlarged, with many additions, and the dose most exactly directed to every medicine. 1852. By A. Gerald Hull, M. D. $1 50.

LAURIE, Dr. J., ELEMENTS OF HOMŒOPATHIC PRACTICE OF PHYSIC. An Appendix to Laurie's Domestic, containing also all the Diseases of THE URINARY AND GENITAL ORGANS. Bound, $1 25.

F. HUMPHREYS, M. D., The Cholera and its Homœopathic Treatment. 38 cts.

B. F. JOSLIN, M. D., Homœopathic Treatment of Diarrhœa, Dysentery, Cholera Morbus and Cholera, with Repertories. 50 cts.

C. HERING'S DOMESTIC PHYSICIAN. Fourth American edition, revised, with additions from the author's manuscript of the 7th German edition. Containing the diseases of Females and Children. $2.

Dr. CASPARI'S HOMŒOPATHIC DOMESTIC PHYSICIAN, edited by F Hartmann, M. D., author of "The Acute and Chronic Diseases." Translated from the eighth German edition, and enriched by a Treatise on Anatomy and Physiology, embellished with 30 illustrations. By W. P. Esrey, M. D., with Additions and a Preface, by C. Hering, M. D., containing also a chapter on Mesmerism and Magnetism; directions for patients living some distance from a Homœopathic physician, to describe their symptoms; a Tabular Index of the Medicines and the Diseases in which they are used; and a Sketch of the Biography of Dr. Samuel Hahnemann, the Founder of Homœopathy. Bound, $1 50.

HOMŒOPATHIC COOKERY. Second edition, with additions, by the lady of an American Homœopathic Physician. Designed chiefly for the use of such persons as are under Homœopathic treatment. 50 cents

JOSLIN, B. F., M. D., PRINCIPLES OF HOMŒOPATHIA. In a series of Lectures. Bound, 75 cts.

AN EPITOME OF HOMŒOPATHIC PRACTICE. Compiled chiefly from Jahr, Rückert, Beauvais, Bönninghausen, &c. By J. T. Curtis, M. D., and J. Lillie, M. D. Second enlarged edition. Bound, 50 cts.

LAURIE'S HOMŒOPATHIC DOMESTIC, by A. Gerald Hull, M. D. Small edition, bound, 50 cts.

ED. C. CHEPMELL'S DOMESTIC HOMŒOPATHY, Restricted to its Legitimate Sphere of Practice, together with Rules for Diet and Regimen. First American edition, with Additions by Samuel B. Barlow, M. D. Bound, 50 cts.

HEMPEL'S HOMŒOPATHIC DOMESTIC PHYSICIAN. Bound, 50 cts.

BŒNNINGHAUSEN'S Essay on the Homœopathic Treatment of Intermittent Fevers. Translated and edited by C. J. Hempel, M. D. 38 cts.

EPP'S, Dr. J., DOMESTIC HOMŒOPATHY; or, Rules for the Domestic Treatment of the Maladies of Infants, Children and Adults, &c. Fourth American from the fourth London edition. Edited and enlarged by George W. Cook, M. D. Bound, 75 cts.

THE FAMILY GUIDE TO THE ADMINISTRATION OF HOMŒOPATHIC REMEDIES. 5th edition after the 3d London edition, by H. V. Malan, M. D.; with additions. 1852. Price 25 cts.

POCKET HOMŒOPATHIST, AND FAMILY GUIDE. By J. A. Tarbell, M. D. Bound 25 cts.

JAHR, G. H. G., M. D., Short Elementary Treatise upon Homœopathia, and the Manner of its Practice; with some of the most important effects of ten of the principal Homœopathic Remedies, for the use of all honest men who desire to convince themselves by experiment of the truth of the doctrine. Second French edition, corrected and enlarged. Translated by Edward Bayard, M. D. Bound, 38 cts.

SHERRIL'S MANUAL OF HOMŒOPATHIC PRESCRIPTION, with an improved Repertory; also an introduction in which the doctrine and nature of the Homœopathic system is explained. 25 cts.

MARINER'S PHYSICIAN AND SURGEON; or a Guide to the Homœopathic Treatment of those diseases to which Seamen are liable. By George W. Cook, M. D. Bound, 38 cts.

J. A. TARBELL, M. D. Sources of Health and Prevention of Disease. 50 cts.

A TREATISE ON THE USE OF ARNICA, in cases of Contusions, Wounds, Sprains, Lacerations of the Solids, Concussions, Paralysis, Rheumatism, Soreness of the Nipples, &c., &c., with a number of cases illustrative of the use of that drug. By Charles Julius Hempel, M. D. 19 cts.

DISEASES OF FEMALES AND CHILDREN. By Walter Williamson, M. D., Professor af Materia Medica, &c., in the Homœopathic Medical College at Philadelphia. Bound, 38 cts.

BECKER, M. D., on Consumption. Translated from the German. 38 cts.

——— on Diseases of the Eye. Translated from the German. 38 cts.

——— on Constipation. Translated from the German. 38 cts.

——— on Dentition. Translated from the German. 38 cts.

——— on Consumption, Diseases of the Eye, Constipation, and Dentition, (containing all four of the above works), bound in one vol. $1.

WM. HENDERSON, M. D., HOMŒOPATHIC PRACTICE. 50 cts.

FORBES, M. D., HOMŒOPATHY, ALLOPATHY, AND YOUNG PHYSIC. 25 cts.

WM. HENDERSON, M. D., LETTER TO J. FORBES. 25 cts.

☞ The above three works bound in 1 vol. $1.

HAHNEMANN'S ORGANON OF HOMŒOPATHIC MEDICINE. 3d American edition, with improvements and additions from the last German edition, and Dr. C. Hering's Introductory Remarks. Bound, $1.

HAHNEMANN'S MATERIA MEDICA PURA. Translated by C. J. Hempel, M. D. 4 vols. $6.

E. STAPF'S ADDITIONS to the Materia Medica Pura. Translated by C. J. Hempel, M. D. $1 50.

HAHNEMANN'S CHRONIC DISEASES, their Specific Nature aud Homœopathic Treatment. Translated and edited by Charles J. Hempel, M. D., with a Preface by Constantine Hering, M. D. 8vo. 5 vols. Bound. $7.

HAHNEMANN'S LESSER WRITINGS, Collected and Translated by R. E. Dudgeon, M. D., with additions by E. E. Marcy, M. D., author of "The Homœopathic Theory and Practice of Medicine," and Editor of the North American Homœopathic Journal." A large 8vo. volume, with a fine steel engraving of S. Hahnemann. 1852. Bound. $3.

☞ The above *five standard* works of Dr. SAMUEL HAHNEMANN are and will FOR EVER be the greatest treasures of Homœopathy; they are the most necessary books for Physicians, and they should grace the library of every lover of science.

Just Published:

LAURIE'S ELEMENTS OF HOMŒOPATHIC PRACTICE OF PHYSIC, by Dr. J. Laurie, with additions by A. G. Hull, M. D., and an Appendix on Intermittent Fevers, by Dr. F. S. Douglas. A large thick 8vo. vol. 1853. $3.

JAHR'S and POSSART'S New Manual of the Homœopathic Materia Medica, containing the characteristic, pathogenetic and curative symptoms of all the principal remedies used in Homœopathic practice; with a Repertory, indicating the remedies which should be used in every single case. Translated and edited by Charles J. Hempel, M. D. 1853. Bound, $4.

MADDEN, HENRY R., M. D., UTERINE DISEASES, with an Appendix containing abstracts of 180 Cases of Uterine Diseases and their treatment, together with Analytical Tables of Results, Ages, Symptoms, Dose, &c., to which is added a Clinical Record of interesting cases treated in the Manchester Homœopathic Hospital. 1852. 50 cts.

RUECKERT ON NERVOUS HEADACHE. Successful Homœopathic Cures, collected from the best homœopathic periodicals, translated and edited by J. C. Peters, M. D. With full descriptions of the dose to each single case. 1853. Bound. 75 cts.

MARCY, E. E., M. D., HOMŒOPATHY AND ALLOPATHY. An Examination of the Doctrines and Evidences of Homœopathy. By Worthington Hooker, M. D. By E. E. Marcy, M. D., author of "The Homœopathic Theory and Practice." 1852. Bound 50 cts.

E. E. MARCY, M. D. THE HOMŒOPATHIC THEORY AND PRACTICE OF MEDICINE. Second edition. 1852. Bound, $2.

BRYANT, Dr. J., A POCKET MANUAL, or Repertory of Homœopathic Medicine, alphabetically and nosologically arranged; which may be used as the physician's Vade-Mecum, the traveller's Medical Companion, or the Family Physician: containing the principal remedies for the most important diseases, symptoms, sensations, characteristics of diseases, &c.; with the principal pathogenetic effects of the medicines on the most important organs and functions of the body; together with diagnosis, explanation of technical terms, directions for the selection and exhibition of the remedies, rules of diet, &c., &c. Compiled from the best authorities. Bound. $1 25.

JAHR'S and GRUNER'S NEW HOMŒOPATHIC PHARMACOPIÆ AND POSOLOGY, or the mode of preparing Homœopathic Medicine, and the Administration of Doses. Compiled and translated from the German works of Buchner, Gruner, and the French work of Jahr, by C. J. Hempel, M. D. Bound, $2.

JAHR'S DISEASES OF THE SKIN; or Alphabetical Repertory of the Skin Symptoms and External Alterations of Substance, together with the morbid phenomena observed in the glandular, osseous, mucous and circulatory systems, arranged with pathological remarks on the Diseases of the Skin. By Dr. A. G. Jahr. Edited by C. J. Hempel, M. D. Price $1.

JAHR'S CLINICAL GUIDE; or Pocket Repertory. Translated from the German, by Charles J. Hempel, M. D. Bound, $1 50.

RUOFF'S REPERTORY OF HOMŒOPATHIC MEDICINE, nosologically arranged. Translated from the German by A. H. Okie, M. D., translator of Hartmann's Remedies. Second American edition, with additions and improvements, by G. Humphrey, M. D., &c. $1 50.

HARTMANN'S ACUTE AND CHRONIC DISEASES, and their Homœopathic Treatment. Third German edition, revised and considerably enlarged by the author. Translated, with additions, and adapted to the use of the American profession, by C. J. Hempel, M. D. 4 vols. $5 75.

HARTMANN, Dr. F., Practical Observations on the two chief Homœopathic remedies of *Belladonna* and *Nux vomica*. By A. H. Okie, M. D. Bound. 50 cts.

TRANSACTIONS of the American Institute of Homœopathy. Or Manual of the New Medicines, tried and arranged by Drs. C. Hering, W. Williamson, C. Neidhard, J. Jeanes, S. Dubs, and J. Kitchen. With a Repertory by W. P. Esrey, M. D. Bound. $1 50.

G. L. RAU'S ORGANON OF THE SPECIFIC HEALING ART OF HOMŒOPATHY. By C. J. Hempel, M. D. $1 25.

HOMŒOPATHIC TREATMENT OF DISEASES OF THE SEXUAL SYSTEM, being a complete Repertory of all the symptoms occurring in the Sexual Systems of the Male and Female. Adapted to the use of physicians and laymen. Translated, arranged and edited, with additions and improvements, by F. Humphreys, M. D. Bound. 50 cts.

HEMPEL'S BŒNNINGHAUSEN for Homœopathic Physicians; to be used at the bedside of the patient, and in studying the Materia Medica Pura. 1 octavo vol., most complete edition, including the Concordances of Homœopathic Remedies. Translated and adapted to the use of the American profession, by C. J. Hempel, M. D. Bound. $2.

www.ingramcontent.com/pod-product-compliance
Lightning Source LLC
LaVergne TN
LVHW011233110826
845150LV00006B/1629

* 9 7 8 1 4 2 5 5 1 4 4 1 9 *